Green Protein

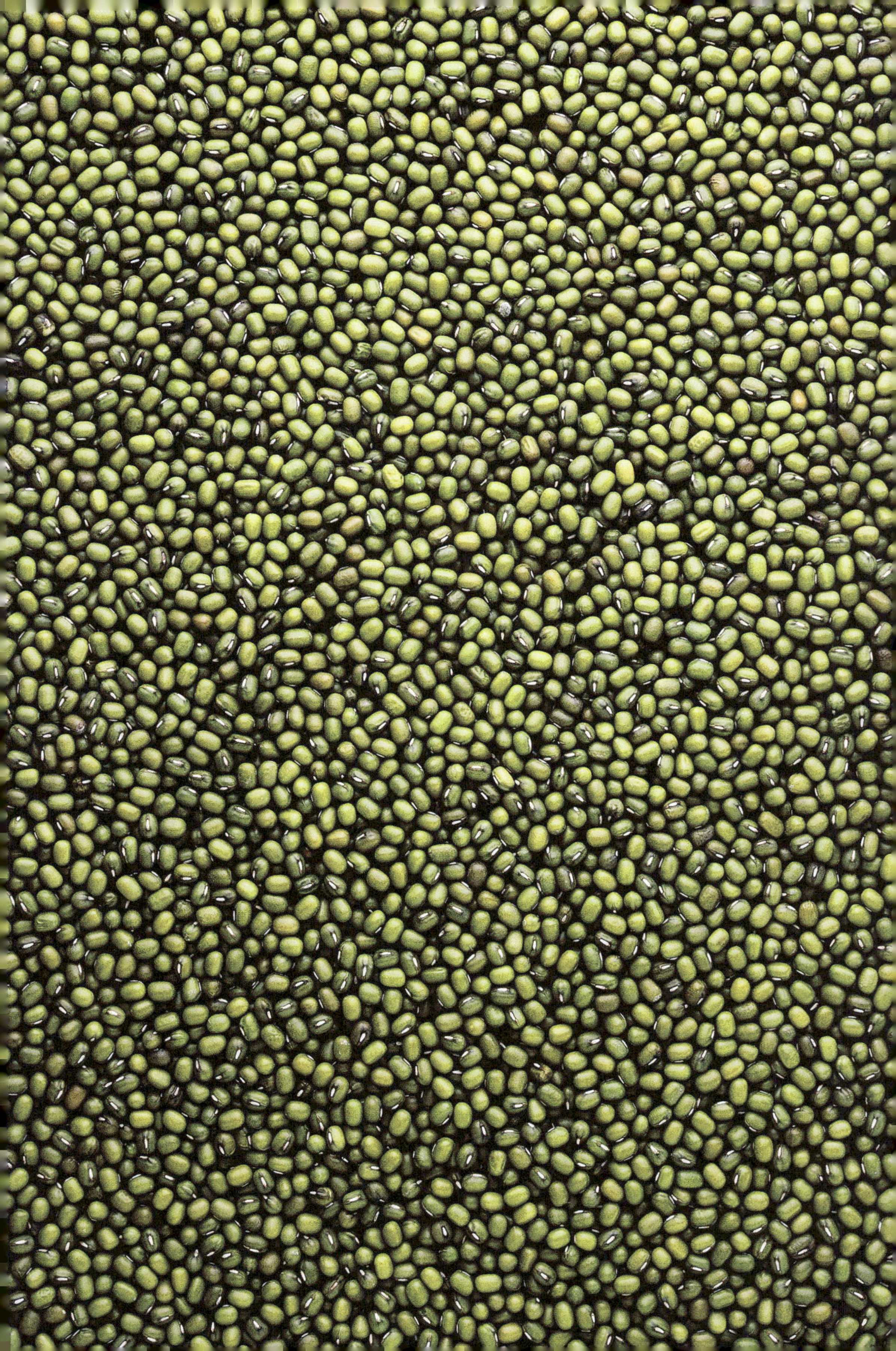

Green Protein

75 ingenious vegan recipes with the extra protein kick

REBEKKA TRUNZ

GRUB STREET • LONDON

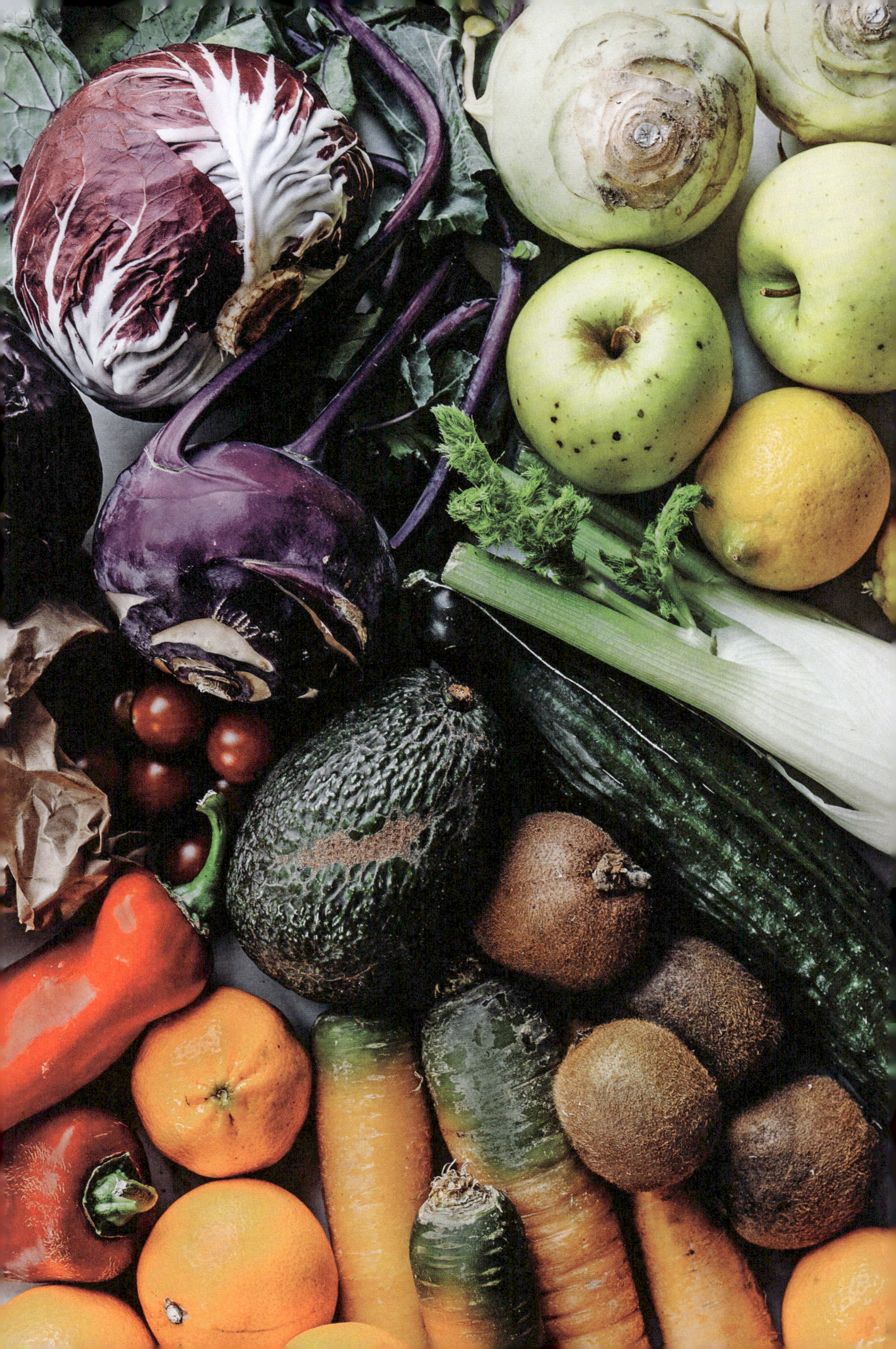

CONTENTS

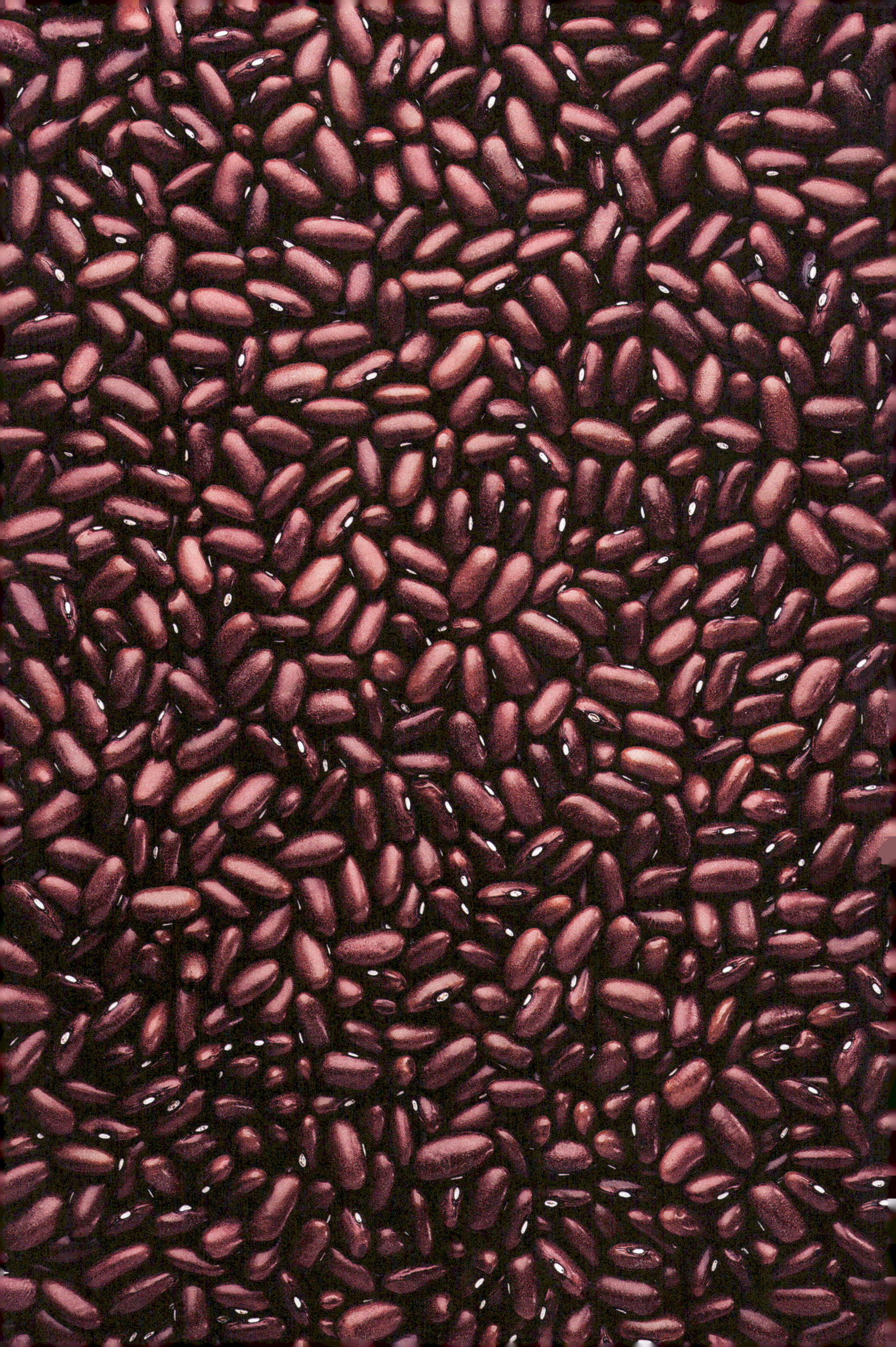

INTRODUCTION

Health reasons, ethical concerns and respect for animals and the environment are some of the many arguments in favour of a plant-based diet. But can our protein requirements be covered by plant-based foods alone? This question is asked by practically everybody deciding to adopt a vegetarian or plant-based diet, or a fully vegan lifestyle, to which the answer is (more or less) surprising. The following pages provide a brief introduction to the world of proteins and everything you need to know about it.

WHAT IS PROTEIN?

The word 'protein' is derived from the Greek *proteios*, which means 'primary'. This name does more than just suggest the importance of this substance; it points to the crucial role that protein compounds, or proteins, play in the human body. Proteins are aptly known as the 'building blocks of life', because nothing in our body would work without them. They play a major part in the body's formation and upkeep, and they determine the structure, function and metabolism of all its cells. Not only do they serve as building material for muscles, tissue and bones, but they're also structural components of enzymes, hormones and the body's immune system.

THE STRUCTURE OF PROTEINS

Proteins are made up of different amino acids. There are 20 known proteinogenic amino acids (required by the human body for protein synthesis), eight of which our body is unable to produce by itself and are known as 'essential', or 'indispensable', amino acids. Essential amino acids must be supplied by our diet. Practically all natural foods contain proteins, but each type of protein has a different amino acid pattern.

EVALUATING PROTEIN QUALITY

How efficiently the proteins in food can be converted into the body's own proteins is determined by their biological value. This is a measure of protein quality in terms of how readily the digested food proteins can be used by the body in protein synthesis. The more similar the amino acid composition of a protein is to that of the human body, the higher its biological value. The quality of any food protein is determined by the least abundant essential amino acid in the protein relative to the body's requirement, which is known as the limiting amino acid. If we make up for this deficient amino acid by adding another food protein, the amino acid patterns complement each other and the biological value of the proteins increases as a result. In addition to biological value, other methods have been established for assessing protein quality, for example, the protein digestibility-corrected amino acid score (PDCAAS) method, which takes into account the digestibility of proteins and determines their actual nutritional value.

THE COMBINATION IS WHAT COUNTS

To meet our daily protein intake requirements (0.75 g of protein per kilogram of body weight according to the British Nutrition Foundation guidelines), the amount of total protein we consume is actually less important than how we combine proteins. Plant proteins usually have an incomplete amino acid profile as they typically lack one or more essential amino acids. However, if we eat a varied, calorie-adequate diet that combines different protein sources, we won't need to worry so much about not achieving the full protein intake. Legumes, for example (which are low in the amino acid methionine and high in lysine), can be ideally complemented by cereals (high in methionine and low in lysine). In combination, they form a complete protein that provides our body with all the amino acids it requires for protein synthesis.

GENERAL FORMULA
Cereals, nuts or seeds
+ legumes
= complete protein

There's no need to combine different protein sources within a single meal. As the body is able to store amino acids for some time, it's sufficient to consider your protein intake spread throughout the day. If you start with a bowl of muesli in the morning, your body will still be able to benefit from tofu in the evening. Basically, protein synthesis can be likened to our body putting together a different three-dimensional jigsaw puzzle every day. All we have to do is provide it with the right building blocks.

EXAMPLES OF SUITABLE FOOD COMBINATIONS (COMPLETE PROTEINS)

- Porridge/muesli with soya milk
- Wholemeal bread with peanut butter
- Dal with rice
- Hummus with pitta
- Pasta with lentil ragù
- Kitchari (mung beans and rice)

Certain plants already have a naturally occurring complete amino acid profile. They include:

- Quinoa
- Buckwheat
- Soya beans
- Lupin beans
- Hemp seeds
- Chia seeds
- Spirulina

ANIMAL PROTEIN VERSUS PLANT PROTEIN

When considered on their own, animal proteins have a higher biological value because they're structurally more similar to human protein. However, they contain a high proportion of saturated fatty acids and cholesterol, which can lead to increased cholesterol levels and favour the development of cardiovascular disease, type 2 diabetes and cancer. On the other hand, not only are plant-based protein sources low in fat and cholesterol-free, but they're also packed with healthy ingredients. They provide plenty of minerals, trace elements, vitamins and healthy fats, as well as complex carbohydrates and fibre. They also contain numerous secondary plant compounds that have a wide range of health benefits for our bodies. This makes plant-based foods both a healthy and nutritious alternative to animal products and a natural form of protection against diseases characteristic of Western civilisation. What's more, what we serve on our plates isn't only important for our own health but also for the health of our planet. Plant proteins can nourish far more people than the same amount of animal proteins. Whether in terms of water consumption, environmental impact or land use, there are immense resource savings associated with a plant-based diet. Satisfying your protein requirements with predominantly plant-based sources is good for your health and significantly contributes to a better and more sustainable future.

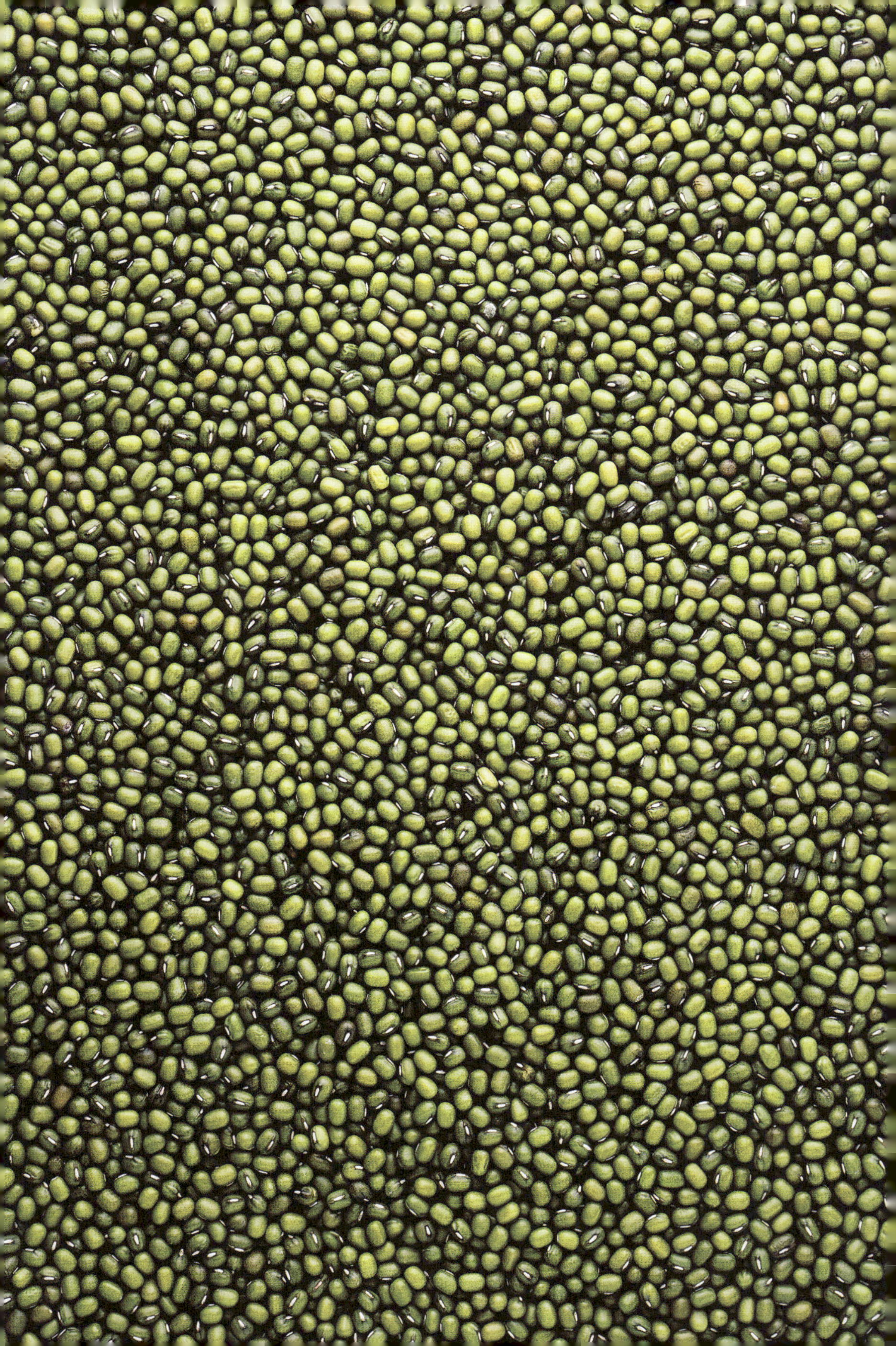

GREEN PROTEIN

When we take a closer look at the plant kingdom, we can see that it's teeming with little powerhouses, and not only do they provide high-quality protein but also plenty of other vital nutrients. Plus, plant-based foods are both satisfying and provide exactly what everybody needs.

Note: All the nutritional information given in the following chapter is based on average values that are subject to natural fluctuations and may vary depending on the plant variety, growing method and the way in which it is processed and/or prepared, among others. The protein content, which is stated in grams (g), refers to 100 g of the particular legume, cereal, vegetable, etc.

LEGUMES

Legumes are plants from the *Fabaceae* (or *Leguminosae*) family, which produce seeds in pods. They're among the oldest and most diverse cultivated plants and have played a major part in human nutrition since Neolithic times. They come in every conceivable shape and colour. Among the most representative examples are pulses, mature and dry seeds that include lentils, dried beans, chickpeas and split peas; tender pods and seeds, considered vegetables, such as green beans and garden peas; and soya beans and peanuts. Legumes are an excellent source of protein and have a high nutritional value. Despite being low in calories, they contain a variety of minerals, trace elements, vitamins and secondary plant compounds. Their fibre and complex carbohydrates keep you full for longer, stabilise blood sugar levels and improve digestion. There's a saying that goes: 'every little bean makes a little noise.'

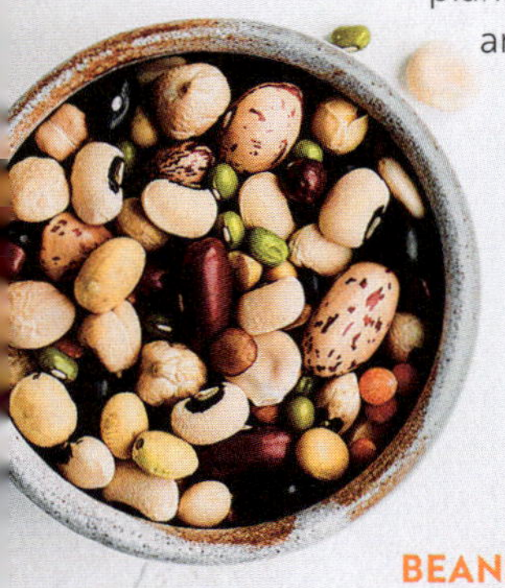

BEANS WITHOUT THE NOISE

The flatulence-inducing effect of legumes, particularly pulses, is mainly due to the complex sugars (oligosaccharides) they contain, which release gases as they break down in the intestine. There are a few things you can do to remove some of these sugars in order to reduce this effect:

Soaking and cooking: Part of the complex sugars in pulses dissolve when soaked and cooked in water. Therefore, it's important to always rinse the pulses well before use and discard both the soaking and cooking water.

Sprouting: Carbohydrates break down during the germination process, which means that the body has to work less in making them more digestible.

Seasoning appropriately: Certain spices, such as caraway seeds, cumin, fennel seeds, aniseed, pepper and ginger contain active ingredients that can prevent flatulence and alleviate its symptoms.

Choosing more digestible varieties: The outer layer, or hull, of pulses mainly comprises insoluble fibre, which is why hulled varieties are easier to digest.

Gradual adaptation: Intestinal flora needs time to adapt to the complex sugars and fibre in pulses. After some time, your intestines are colonised by microorganisms that are better suited to metabolising their compounds.

WHAT'S INSIDE?

Red lentils (25.9 g), like yellow lentils, aren't actually a variety of lentil in the true sense but mostly hulled and split brown lentils. This not only gives them a more colourful appearance but also makes them less complicated to prepare and easier to digest.

Brown lentils (23.4 g) are comparatively large, with a diameter of 6–7 millimetres. Their nutty, slightly earthy flavour makes them a popular ingredient for soups and rustic stews. Depending on how they are stored, their colour can range from greenish brown to yellowish brown.

Beluga lentils (23.4 g), also known as caviar lentils, get their name from their appearance, as these small, black and shiny lentils resemble beluga caviar.

Peas (5.4 g, fresh) come in different varieties, both fresh and dried. A distinction is made between dried (marrowfat and split) peas, garden (fresh) peas and mangetout.

Chickpeas (19 g) originated in the Middle East, where they were first cultivated over 8,000 years ago. Hummus and falafel would be completely unthinkable without these pulses. Did you know that chickpeas aren't just yellow-orange, and that they can also be brown or black?

Green beans (2.4 g, fresh), also known as French beans, is the collective term for all varieties of bush (dwarf) and pole (runner) beans that are picked immature in the pod and eaten together with it.

Kidney beans (24.2 g) are so-called because of their shape, which unmistakeably resembles that of a kidney. These slightly sweet and somewhat mealy beans are mainly grown in Africa and the Americas.

Adzuki beans (20.9 g) originated in Japan, where they are used to make many traditional desserts, including mochi, glutinous rice flour cakes that are filled with a sweet paste made from these beans.

Pinto beans (21 g) have a particularly lovely appearance. 'Pinto' means 'painted' in Spanish, which refers to their speckling.

Mung beans (23.1 g) are widely used in Chinese and Indian cuisines and are known for their mild, nutty flavour. They can be prepared in many different ways: hulled or unhulled, whole or split, and cooked or as sprouts.

Black-eyed beans (23.5 g), also known as black-eyed peas, originated in Africa, where they are a popular ingredient in stews and curries. The name of this cowpea subspecies comes from its distinctive black spot.

Black beans (23.1 g), also known as black turtle beans, are native to South and Central America and are a staple of Latin American cuisine. They're now also becoming increasingly popular in Europe.

Soya beans (37.6 g) are given a special place among legumes owing to their nutritional value. In addition to their high fat content, they provide plenty of high-quality protein that contains all the essential amino acids. This makes soya beans ideal for making different dairy and meat substitutes, as well as for tofu, tempeh, etc.

Edamame (11.7 g, fresh) are unripe soya beans picked in their pods, which are typically served as a snack in many Japanese restaurants. Their Japanese name means 'stem beans'.

Lupin beans (43 g) are high in fibre and micronutrients, as well as high-quality protein, making them a good local alternative to mostly imported soya beans.

Peanuts (25.3 g), also known as ground nuts, don't belong to the botanical nut family, despite their name. They actually belong to the legume family, like beans and peas.

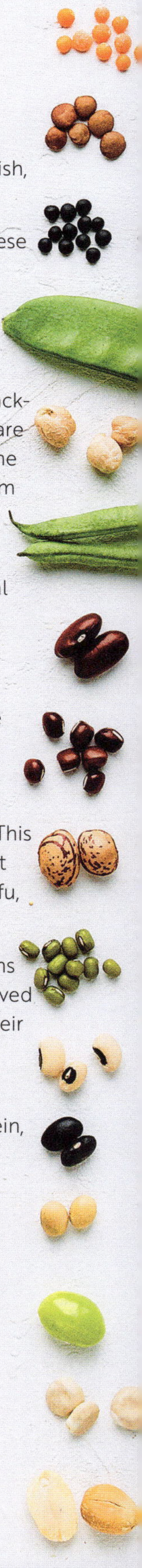

CEREALS & PSEUDOCEREALS

Cereals have been one of our most important staple foods for thousands of years. Whether in the form of bread, pasta, muesli or grains, they have become an integral part of our diet. These small grains largely consist of complex carbohydrates and provide us with plenty of plant protein, valuable minerals, essential vitamins and fibre, which aids intestinal transit and helps to build up our intestinal flora. You should always choose wholegrain cereals, as they contain the most nutrients. There are seven major varieties of true cereals (grasses): wheat, barley, rye, oats, maize, millet and rice.

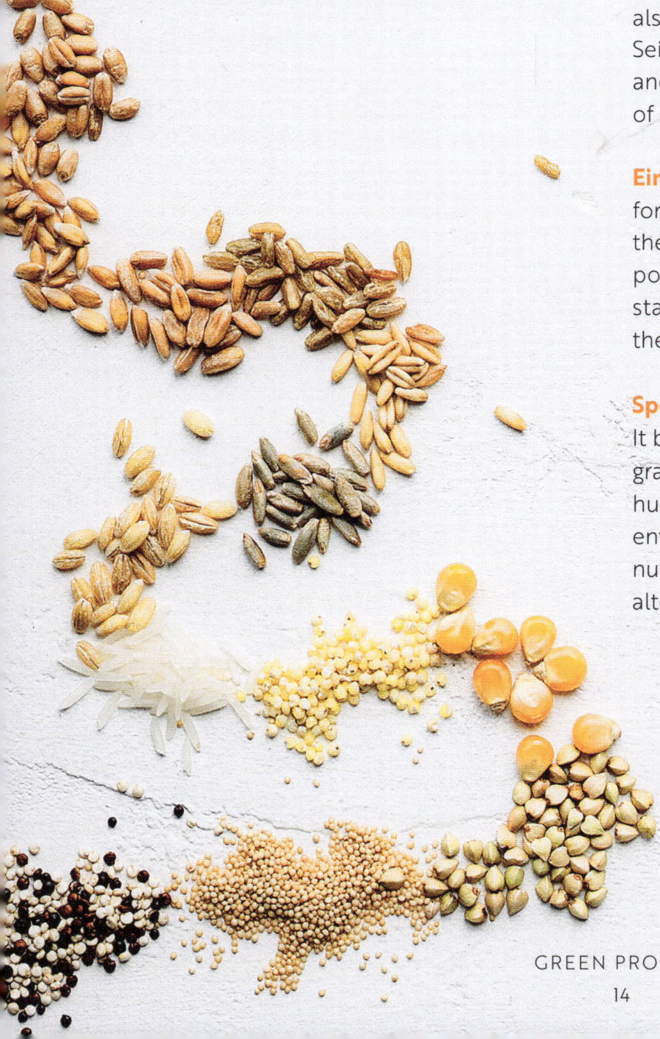

Grains that resemble cereals in appearance and use but aren't produced by grasses are known as pseudocereals. These include buckwheat, quinoa, canihua (also known as kañiwa or baby quinoa) and amaranth – they're all gluten-free and are considered superfoods.

WHAT'S INSIDE?

Wheat (11.4 g) is the best known and most important cereal in use today. Its white flour is used to make bread, cakes and pastries, and it's also an ingredient of various breakfast cereals. Seitan is made from pure wheat protein (gluten) and serves as a base for making a wide variety of meat substitutes.

Einkorn (15.9 g) and emmer are the earliest forms of domesticated wheat, which is why they are also known as ancient grains. They possess a number of nutritional benefits and stand out from ordinary cereals because of their particularly high nutrient content.

Spelt (13.2 g) is closely related to modern wheat. It belongs to the group of husked cereals whose grain is surrounded by a protective coating, the husk or hull, that protects it from pests and environmental conditions. Due to its higher nutrient density, spelt makes an excellent alternative to wheat.

Green spelt (11.4 g) is spelt that is harvested at an early stage and then dried and roasted. With its nutty and smoky flavour, it's perfect for rustic stews, soups and rissoles.

Barley (10.4 g) is mostly found in the form of flakes, flour, groats and pearl barley. It's also the main grain used to make malt, an important ingredient in beer, whisky and malted drinks.

Rye (8.8 g) contains comparatively little protein, but it has the most fibre of all cereals, as well as plenty of vitamins and minerals.

Oats (12.5 g) are among the cereals with the highest protein content, and have the most fat and minerals of all of them, especially iron and calcium. In the form of porridge oats, they have definitely earned a permanent place on the shopping list. They're perfect for a balanced and healthy breakfast.

Maize (8.5 g) was originally brought from Mexico to Europe by Christopher Columbus. Alongside wheat and rice, it is one of the most widely grown cereal crops today. Yellow sweetcorn can be cooked or the kernels nibbled straight off the cob.

Millet (9.8 g) is characterised above all by its high iron content, which is far higher than that of other cereals. In addition to golden millet, there is also the darker browntop millet and teff (dwarf millet), the world's smallest grain.

Basmati rice (7.2 g) is one of the best-known types of rice. Basmati means 'fragrant', which is already an indication of its delicate flavour. Mainly grown in the foothills of the Himalayas, basmati rice is a typical accompaniment for Indian and Middle Eastern dishes.

Quinoa (13.8 g) was already a staple food for the Inca civilisation. Quinoa grains, which are the size of mustard seeds, are high in valuable protein and contain iron, potassium and other nutrients.

Amaranth (14.6 g) gets its name from the Greek word *amarantos*, which means 'undying'. These small grains contain considerable amounts of calcium, magnesium, iron and zinc. Its high protein content makes amaranth a veritable dynamo.

Buckwheat (9.1 g), which belongs to the knotweed family, has a distinctive nutty flavour.
In addition to different essential nutrients, these triangular grains provide us with high-quality protein that contains all the amino acids we need.

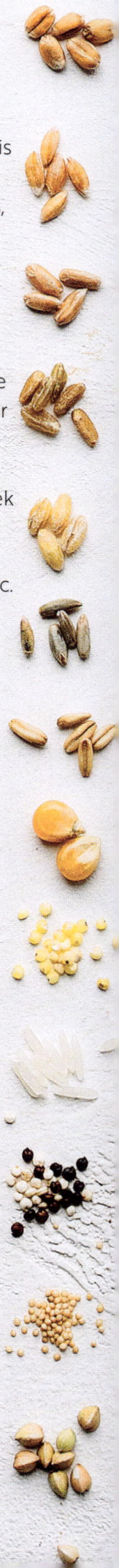

NUTS & SEEDS

Because of their high fat content, nuts and seeds have comparatively high calorie count. Doesn't that make them less healthy? In fact, the opposite is true. These little powerhouses are rich in healthy fats and high-quality plant protein. They provide us with a wide range of valuable minerals, such as potassium, magnesium, zinc and phosphorus, as well as essential vitamins – B-group vitamins and vitamin E, in particular. They also contain plenty of fibre, antioxidants and secondary plant compounds. Their high content in monounsaturated and polyunsaturated fatty acids means a great deal of positive effects on our physical and mental health. Eaten regularly as part of a balanced and healthy diet, nuts lower cholesterol and triglyceride levels, protect our heart and reduce the risk of cardiovascular disease and cancer. Epidemiological studies also show that they have a positive influence on our body weight and can help with weight loss. Isn't that good to hear?

WHAT'S INSIDE?

Walnuts (14.4 g) have an optimal ratio of omega-6 to omega-3 fatty acids and are particularly rich in alpha-linolenic acid, an essential fatty acid that produces a range of positive effects on our health and well-being.

Hazelnuts (12 g) should not be missing from any trail mix. Not only do they make a tasty snack between meals, but their valuable components also nourish nerves and improve memory.

Almonds (18.7 g) are packed with protein. According to studies, 30–60 g of almonds a day are enough to protect us from diabetes, cardiovascular disease and high cholesterol. Almonds aren't true nuts in the botanical sense but the seeds of a stone fruit, like apples and peaches.

Pistachio nuts (20.8 g), in addition to their striking green colour, are also remarkably beneficial to our health. They provide valuable protein, as well as large amounts of potassium, phosphorus, B-group vitamins and vitamin A.

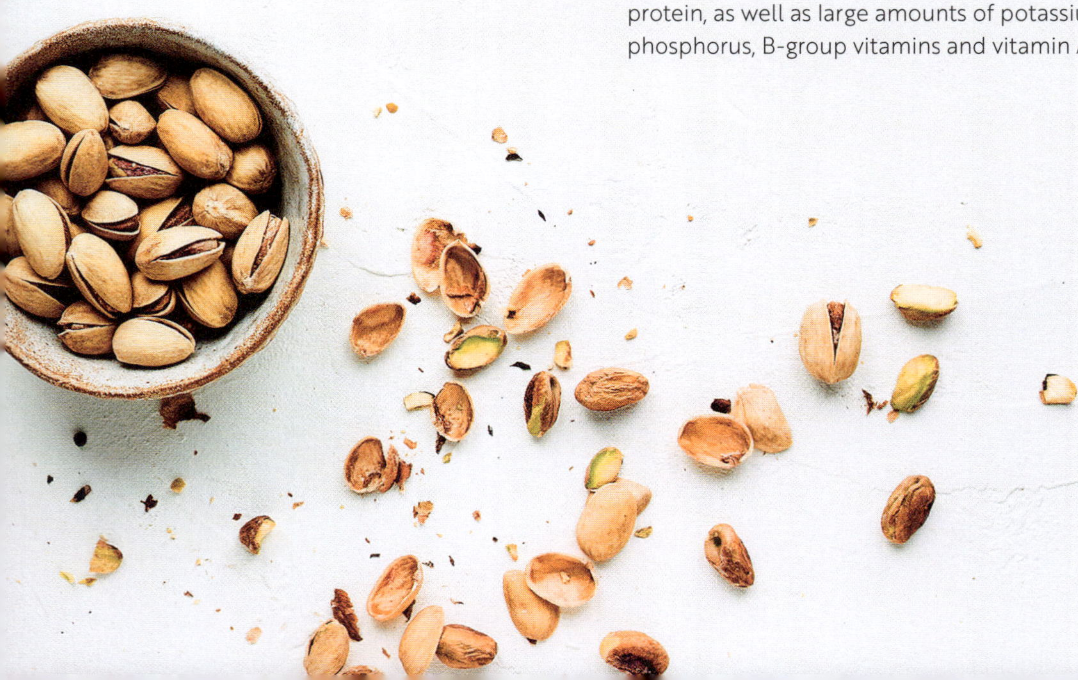

Brazil nuts (13.6 g) are particularly high in fat. However, they contain more selenium than any other plant-based food. Depending on the selenium content of the soil where they were grown, just one or two Brazil nuts can cover our daily requirement of this important trace element.

Cashew nuts (17.2 g) are the seeds of the cashew apple, a fruit resembling a red pepper. The kidney-shaped seeds don't ripen inside the fruit, but hang from the bottom. They have a delicate, slightly sweet flavour.

Pumpkin seeds (24.4 g) are bursting with nutrients. Not only do they contain considerable amounts of plant protein, but they also provide a range of valuable fatty acids, vitamins and minerals, such as iron, magnesium, potassium and phosphorus.

Sunflower seeds (22.5 g) contain a balanced mix of micro and macronutrients. The fat they contain consists of 90 per cent heart-healthy fatty acids, making them an ideal addition to any diet.

Hemp seeds (30 g) provide plenty of high-quality protein that include all essential amino acids, as well as valuable fatty acids, minerals, vitamins and antioxidants. However, eating these seeds won't make you high because they don't contain the intoxicating tetrahydrocannabinol (THC) compound.

Linseed (24.4 g), also known as flaxseed, is rich in fibre and swells significantly in contact with liquid. Its high content in monounsaturated and polyunsaturated fatty acids makes it a veritable superfood.

Sesame seeds (17.7 g) may be small, but they pack a punch with plenty of protein and valuable minerals, such as iron, calcium and magnesium. They come in both black and white versions.

Chia seeds (16.5 g) were already a staple food of advanced civilisations, such as the Maya and Aztecs. Chia comes from the Mayan language and means 'strength', a reference to the power concentrated in these seeds. Chia seeds also swell significantly on contact with liquid, a property that both benefits intestinal transit and gives them a range of culinary uses.

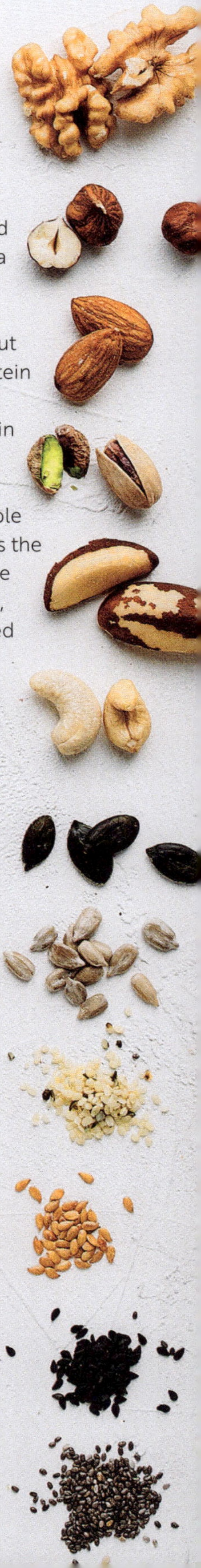

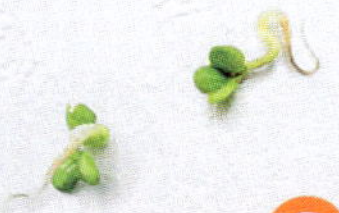

OTHER PLANT-BASED PROTEIN SOURCES

VEGETABLES

As trivial as it may sound, vegetables also provide us with plenty of plant protein. And while they don't have the same concentrations as legumes, cereals, nuts and seeds, seeing as we eat significantly more of them, it all adds up over the course of the day. Vegetables hardly have any calories, which is why we can eat our fill without hesitation and benefit from all their healthy nutrients. Most vegetables provide 1–3 g of protein per 100 g, more or less, and some even more. Green leafy vegetables, such as Brussels sprouts, kale, chard, spinach and broccoli, are particularly noteworthy. A large salad containing steamed broccoli provides a whopping 20 g of protein but only about 150 kilocalories (kcal).

MUSHROOMS

Despite some weird names, like hare's ear, suede bolete and trooping funnel, mushrooms not only contain valuable vitamins and minerals, but they can even be as much as 50 per cent protein. With an average of 20 kcal per 100 g, they're veritable lightweights. King oyster mushrooms and porcini mushrooms are particularly good sources of protein, as are button mushrooms and oyster mushrooms, for example.

SPROUTED SEEDS, SPROUTS & MICROGREENS

The germination process is a miracle of nature. It brings to light the life force that lies dormant in plants. When seeds are soaked in water, a large number of metabolic processes begin after just a few hours. Proteins are converted into amino acids, which not only increases their digestibility but also the number of essential amino acids and, consequently, their biological value. This makes sprouted (germinated) seeds, sprouts (germinated seeds with above-ground shoots) and microgreens (shoots with the first leaves) particularly high-quality sources of protein. What's more, their nutrient content also increases many times over. Fats and anti-nutrients (e.g. protease inhibitors, which inhibit protein breakdown, and phytic acid, which reduces the availability of minerals) are broken down, while valuable vitamins, minerals, trace elements and enzymes are formed. Complex carbohydrates are broken down into simple sugars, which our body digests more easily. Sprouts may be small, but they're packed with plant power and make a healthy, delicious and variable addition to our diet. You can also grow them yourself with little effort. Pulses (e.g. mung beans, lentils and chickpeas), cereals (e.g. spelt, rye and oats), pseudocereals (e.g. buckwheat and quinoa), vegetable seeds (e.g. broccoli, radish, mustard, alfalfa) and nuts and seeds (e.g. almonds, pumpkin seeds and sunflower seeds) are suitable for sprouting.

SEAWEED

With a protein content of up to 70 per cent, seaweed is a marine superfood. It's low in calories, virtually fat-free and bursting with healthy compounds. Although eating large amounts of seaweed on a regular basis isn't recommended, they make a healthy supplement, as well as a tasty ingredient for seafood dishes, soups and salads. A distinction is made between microalgae (unicellular organisms such as spirulina and chlorella) and macroalgae (multicellular organisms, such as nori, wakame, kombu kelp and dulse).

LEGUMES

Adzuki beans	20.9 g*
Alfalfa sprouts, raw	4 g*
Beluga lentils	23.4 g*
Black beans	23.1 g*
Black-eyed beans	23.5 g*
Brown lentils	23.4 g*
Chickpeas	19 g*
Edamame, fresh	11.7 g*
Garden peas, fresh	5.4 g*
Green beans, fresh	2.4 g*
Haricot beans	21.1 g*
Kidney beans	24.2 g*
Lupin groats	42.9 g*
Mung bean sprouts, raw	3.2 g*
Mung beans	23.1 g*
Peanuts	25.3 g*
Pinto beans	21 g*
Red lentils	25.9 g*
Soya beans	37.6 g*
Soya milk	3.6 g*
Soya mince	49 g*
Soya yoghurt	4.8 g*
Tempeh	17.4 g*
Tofu, firm	16 g*

CEREALS & PSEUDOCEREALS

Amaranth	14.6 g*
Buckwheat	9.1 g*
Couscous (durum wheat semolina)	11.3 g*
Green spelt groats	11.4 g*
Millet	9.8 g*
Polenta	8.8 g*
Porridge oats	13.5 g*
Quinoa	13.8 g*
Rice	7.2 g*
Rye	8.8 g*
Spelt	13.2 g*
Sprouted cereal grains, raw	3.2 g*
Wheat	11.4 g*
Wheat protein (gluten)	72 g*
Wholegrain spelt semolina	17 g*

NUTS & SEEDS

Almonds	18.7 g*
Brazil nuts	13.6 g*
Cashew nuts	17.2 g*
Chestnuts	3.4 g*
Chia seeds	16.5 g*
Hazelnuts	12 g*
Hemp seeds	30 g*
Linseed	24.4 g*
Pistachio nuts	20.8 g*
Poppy seeds	20.2 g*
Pumpkin seeds	24.4 g*
Sesame seeds	17.7 g*
Sunflower seeds	22.5 g*
Walnuts	14.4 g*

VEGETABLES

Bamboo shoots	2.5 g*
Broccoli	3.3 g*
Brussels sprouts	4.5 g*
Cauliflower	2.5 g*
Kale	4.3 g*
Potato	2 g*
Savoy cabbage	3 g*
Spinach	2.7 g*

MUSHROOMS

King oyster mushroom	4.4 g*
Oyster mushroom	2.3 g*
Porcini mushroom	5.4 g*
White (button) mushroom	2.7 g*

OTHERS

Nutritional yeast (yeast flakes)	48.1 g*
Nori sheets	48.4 g*
Spirulina	57.5 g*

*Protein per 100 g (edible portion).

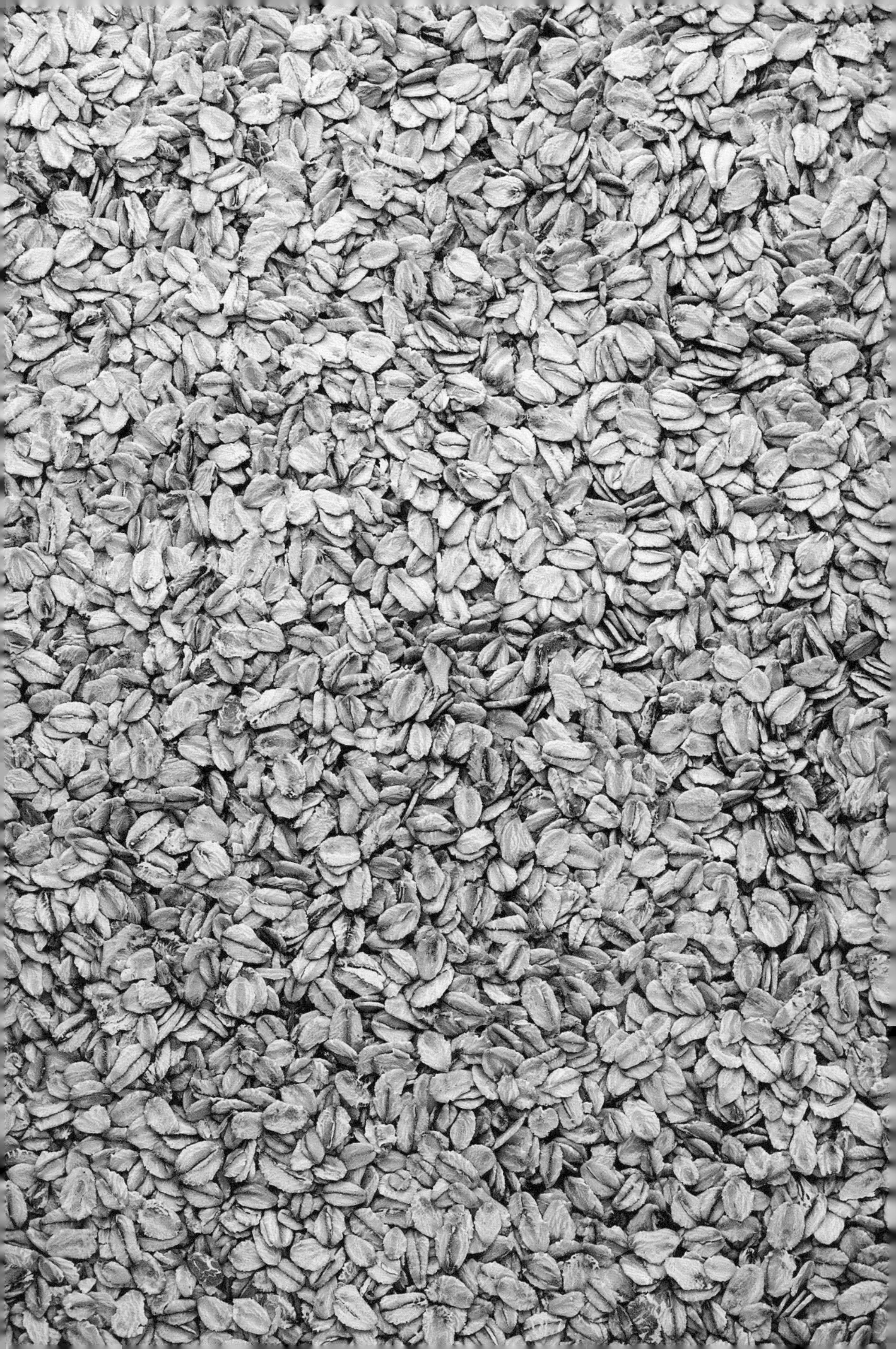

BREAKFAST

A balanced breakfast leaves you full and satisfied, boosts your metabolism and provides you with the energy to get your day off to a good start. Whether you like to take your time and enjoy it with a cup of coffee or tea, or you usually have to eat and run, you're sure to find the right breakfast for you in this section.

OVERNIGHT OATS

4 VERSIONS – SERVES 1

BASIC INGREDIENTS

50 g jumbo porridge oats
1 tbsp chia seeds
150 ml plant-based milk
2 tsp maple syrup (optional)
Toppings of your choice (e.g. berries, chopped nuts, desiccated coconut)

1 PEANUT BUTTER & JELLY OATS

Basic ingredients
1–2 tbsp peanut butter
100 g fresh or frozen (and thawed) raspberries
1 tbsp chia seeds

Mix the basic ingredients together with the peanut butter in a glass. Mix the raspberries and chia seeds in a bowl, then add this mixture to the glass and chill in the fridge overnight. The next morning, serve the overnight oats with toppings of your choice.

2 MIXED BERRY OATS

Basic ingredients
2 tbsp soya yoghurt
1 tbsp ground almonds
100 g fresh or frozen (and thawed) mixed berries

Mix the basic ingredients together with the soya yoghurt, almonds and berries in a glass and chill in the fridge overnight. The next morning, serve the overnight oats with toppings of your choice.

3 MANGO LASSI OATS

Basic ingredients
2 tbsp coconut yoghurt (or substitute with soya yoghurt)
1 tbsp desiccated coconut
100 g mango purée
1 handful diced mango
1 tbsp chia seeds

Mix the basic ingredients together with the coconut yoghurt and desiccated coconut in a glass.
Mix the mango purée, mango cubes and chia seeds together in a bowl, then add this mixture to the glass and chill in the fridge overnight. The next morning, serve the overnight oats with toppings of your choice.

4 CARROT CAKE OATS

Basic ingredients
2 tbsp soya yoghurt
1 tbsp grated carrot
1 tbsp grated apple
1 tbsp chopped walnuts
1 tbsp raisins
1 tsp ground cinnamon

Mix the basic ingredients together with the other ingredients in a glass and chill in the fridge overnight. The next morning, serve the overnight oats with toppings of your choice.

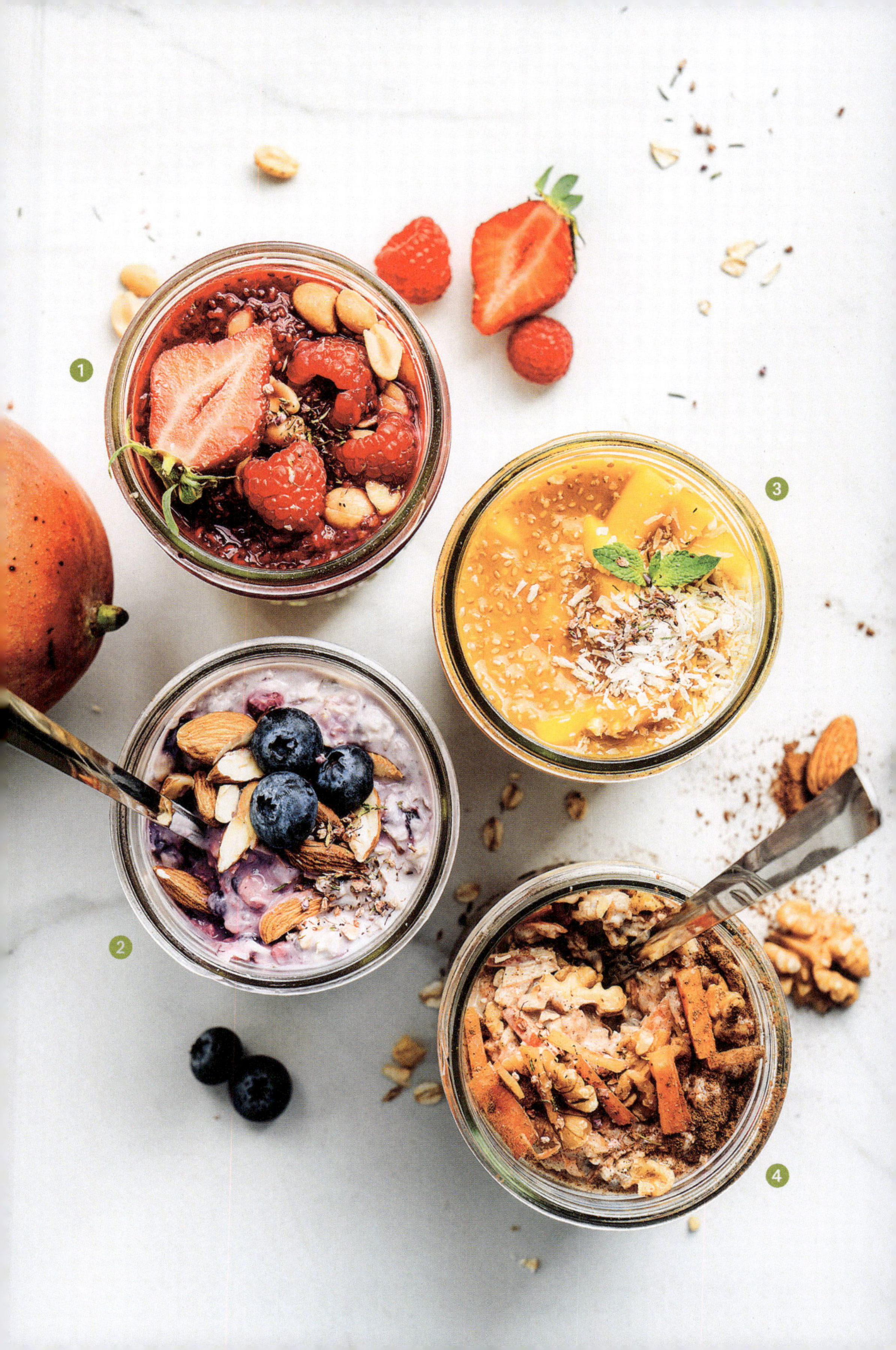
1
2
3
4

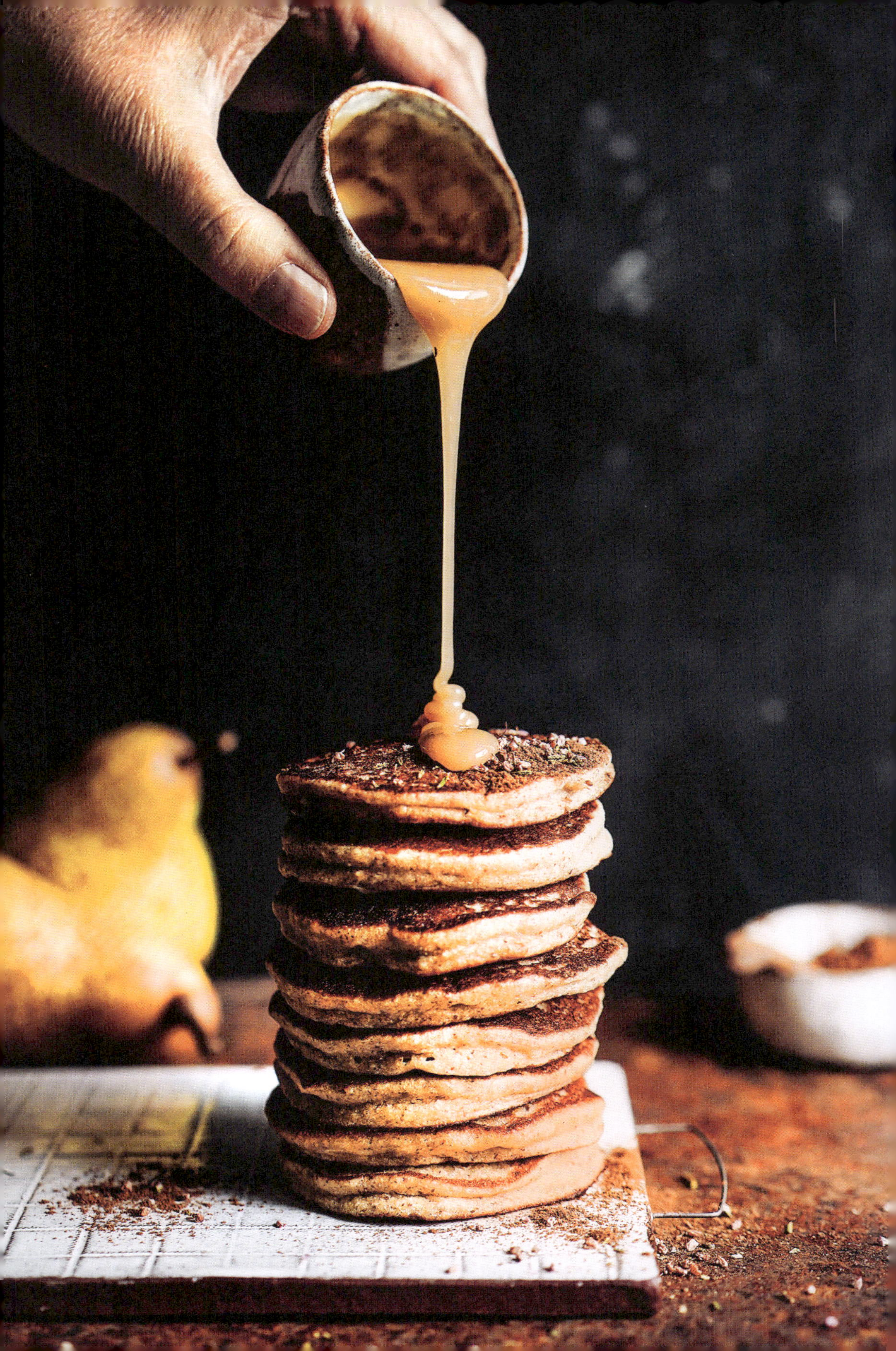

OAT & SPELT PANCAKES WITH COCONUT CARAMEL

SERVES 1

FOR THE COCONUT CARAMEL *(makes 200 ml)*

400 ml coconut milk (at least 60% coconut extract)
100 g raw cane sugar
1 large pinch of sea salt

FOR THE PANCAKES *(makes 8)*

50 g thin-rolled porridge oats
50 g wholemeal spelt flour
1 tbsp Bourbon vanilla sugar
1 tsp baking powder
50 g soya yoghurt (or substitute with apple sauce or 1/2 mashed banana)
125 ml plant-based milk
1 tsp apple cider vinegar
Rapeseed oil for frying

EXTRAS

Fruit of your choice (e.g. pear, apple, banana)
Ground cinnamon

To make the coconut caramel, put the coconut milk into a pan and bring to the boil, then stir in the sugar and salt. Reduce the heat and allow to simmer for 15 minutes, then stir well and reduce for a further 5–10 minutes, until the caramel has thickened just enough to coat the back of a spoon. Transfer the caramel to a screw-top jar while still hot and allow to cool to room temperature.

To make the pancakes, finely grind the oats and mix them with the remaining dry ingredients in a bowl. Add the wet ingredients and mix briefly to a lump-free batter (if it thickens too much, add a little liquid). Heat some oil in a non-stick frying pan and add a heaped tablespoon of batter to the hot pan for each pancake. Cook the pancakes over a medium heat for 1–2 minutes each side, until golden brown.

Serve the pancakes with some coconut caramel and the fruit of your choice. Sprinkle with cinnamon.

• NOTE •

With the lid tightly sealed, the jar of coconut caramel can be stored in the fridge. This will also give it a firmer, spreadable consistency that's absolutely divine on toast. Briefly heating the caramel will turn it back into a sauce. If you prefer a more intense caramel flavour, you can also make this caramel using a darker sugar, such as coconut blossom sugar or whole cane sugar.

WARMING GRAIN PORRIDGE

5 VERSIONS – SERVES 2

1 SIMPLE PORRIDGE

120 g thin-rolled porridge oats
300 ml plant-based milk
2 tbsp ground almonds
2 tsp maple syrup (optional)

Put all the ingredients into a pan, mix with 300 ml of water and bring to the boil. Then reduce the heat and allow to simmer for a few minutes while stirring, until the porridge reaches the desired consistency. Serve with toppings of your choice (e.g. banana, peanut butter).

2 COCONUT RICE PORRIDGE

120 g short-grain pudding rice
150 ml plant-based milk
150 ml coconut milk (at least 60% coconut extract)
2 tbsp desiccated coconut
1–2 tbsp maple syrup (to taste)

Put all the ingredients into a pan, mix with 200 ml of water and bring to the boil. Then reduce the heat to low, cover the pan and allow to simmer for 20 minutes, until the rice is soft. Stir occasionally (more frequently towards the end) to keep from burning. Add a little liquid if necessary. Serve the rice porridge with toppings of your choice (e.g. mango cubes, coconut chips).

3 CHOCOLATE MILLET PORRIDGE

120 g golden millet
300 ml plant-based milk
1 heaped tbsp cocoa powder
1–2 tbsp maple syrup (to taste)
1 pinch of sea salt

Put the millet, plant-based milk and 300 ml of water into a pan and bring to the boil. Then reduce the heat to low, cover the pan and allow to simmer for 15 minutes, stirring from time to time. Stir in the cocoa, maple syrup and salt, then cover the pan, turn off the heat and allow the millet to stand on the still-warm hob for 10 minutes. Serve the chocolate millet porridge with toppings of your choice (e.g. chopped chocolate, berries).

4 SPELT SEMOLINA PORRIDGE

300 ml plant-based milk
80 g spelt semolina
2 tbsp ground almonds
1 tbsp maple syrup

Mix the plant-based milk and 300 ml of water in a pan and bring to the boil. Then remove from the heat and stir in the semolina. Bring everything back to the boil, reduce the heat and cook the semolina for 5 minutes to a porridge consistency, stirring constantly. Turn off the heat, stir in the ground almonds and maple syrup and allow the semolina to stand on the still-warm hob for 10 minutes. Serve with toppings of your choice (e.g. pear, almonds, cinnamon).

5 APPLE AND CINNAMON COUSCOUS PORRIDGE

1 large apple, finely diced
250 ml plant-based milk
120 g couscous
1 tsp ground cinnamon
2 tsp maple syrup (optional)

Put the diced apple and plant-based milk into a pan and bring to the boil. Then stir in the remaining ingredients, turn off the heat and cover the pan. Allow the couscous to stand on the still-warm hob for 10 minutes. Serve with toppings of your choice (e.g. dates, cinnamon).

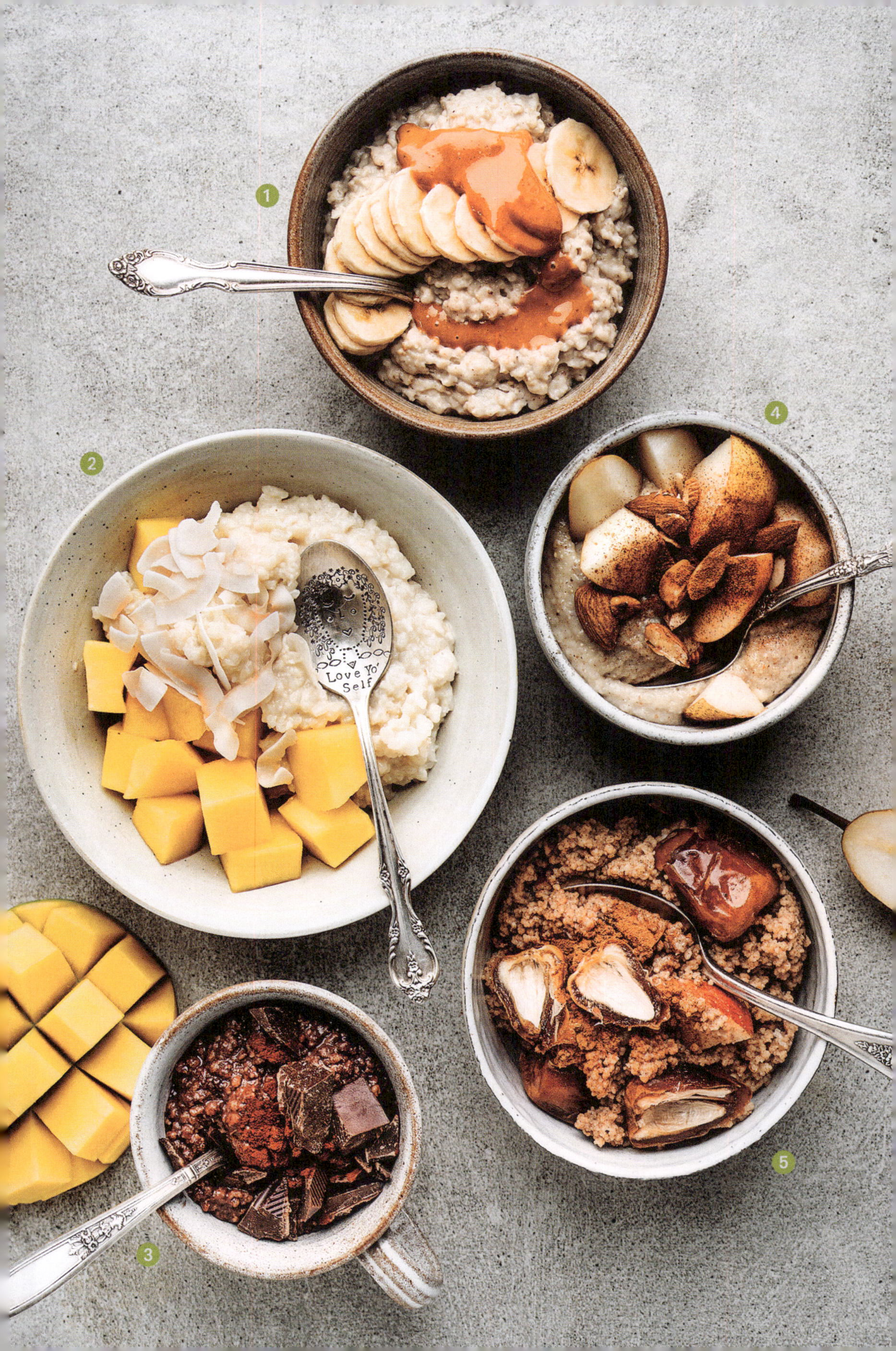
1
2
3
4
5
Love Yo' Self

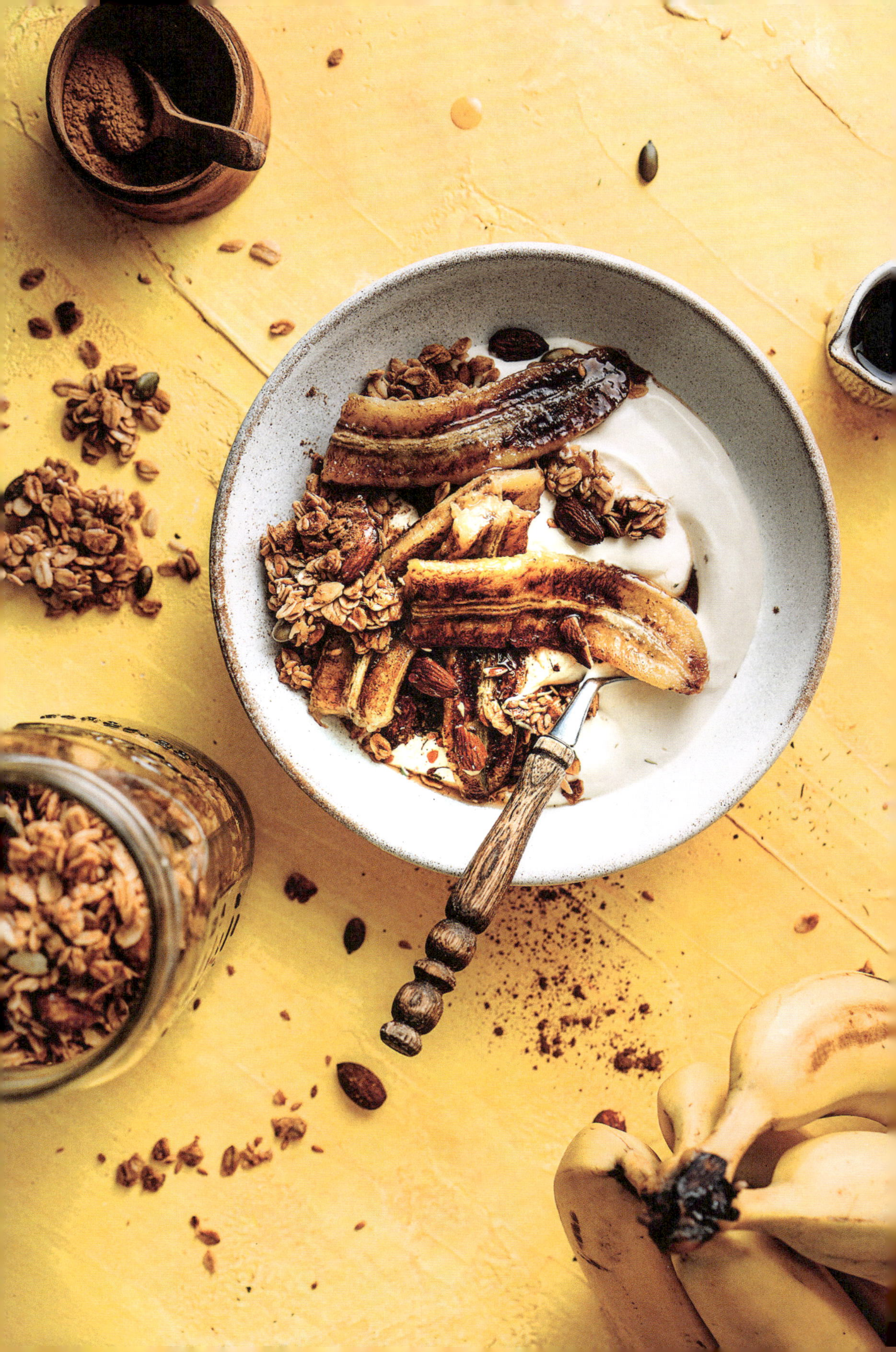

CINNAMON BREAKFAST BOWL

SERVES 2

FOR THE ALMOND AND CINNAMON GRANOLA *(makes 1 tray)*

150 g almonds
250 g jumbo porridge oats
50 g pumpkin seeds
3 tbsp linseed
120 g maple syrup
60 g coconut oil, melted
1 tbsp ground cinnamon

EXTRAS

2 bananas
2 tsp plant-based margarine
2 tbsp maple syrup
400 g soya quark

Preheat the oven to 180°C.

To make the granola, roughly chop half the almonds and mix them together with the oats, pumpkin seeds and linseed in a large bowl. In a small bowl, mix the maple syrup with the coconut oil and add this mixture to the bowl with the oats. Mix well until combined, then spread the mixture over a baking tray lined with baking paper. Bake for 10 minutes, then stir and bake for a further 10–15 minutes (watch closely in the final minutes to keep from burning). Remove the granola from the oven, sprinkle with the cinnamon while still hot and allow to cool to room temperature.

Peel the bananas and slice them in half lengthways. Melt the margarine in a frying pan and stir in the maple syrup. Add the banana halves and fry on both sides until golden brown.

To serve, stir the quark until creamy and divide it between two bowls. Arrange the fried bananas and the almond and cinnamon granola over the quark and serve.

· NOTE ·

Once cooled, you can transfer the granola to a large screw-top jar. With the lid tightly sealed, it can be stored for a few weeks in a dry place. Use it to add a touch of crispy sweetness to any breakfast creation.

CHEESECAKE OATS AND CINNAMON APPLEBAKED IN A SQUASH

SERVES 1

FOR THE SQUASH BOWL

1/2 red kuri squash

FOR THE CHEESECAKE OATS

50 g thin-rolled porridge oats
2 tbsp ground almonds
1 tbsp raisins
150 g soya yoghurt
50 ml plant-based milk
1 tbsp maple syrup
1/2 tsp vanilla extract

FOR THE CINNAMON APPLE TOPPING

1/2 small apple, finely diced
1 tbsp chopped almonds
1 tsp maple syrup
1 tsp ground cinnamon

EXTRAS

Cinnamon sugar

Preheat the oven to 200°C.

To make the bowl, wash the half-squash and scoop out the seeds. Then place it cut-side up on a baking tray lined with baking paper. If it tips over, stand the squash upright in an ovenproof dish. Bake for 30–40 minutes (depending on size), until almost cooked.

To make the cheesecake oats, mix all the dry ingredients together in a bowl, then add the remaining ingredients and mix everything until combined.

To make the cinnamon apple, mix all the ingredients together in a bowl.

After baking for the required time, remove the half-squash from the oven. Fill the squash with cheesecake oats, spread the cinnamon apple over the top and bake again for a further 15 minutes. Remove the squash from the oven, sprinkle the cheesecake oats with cinnamon sugar and serve immediately.

· NOTE ·

These cheesecake oats can also be easily prepared without the squash bowl. In this case, bake the oats into an ovenproof dish for 15 minutes at 200°C heat as described in the recipe.

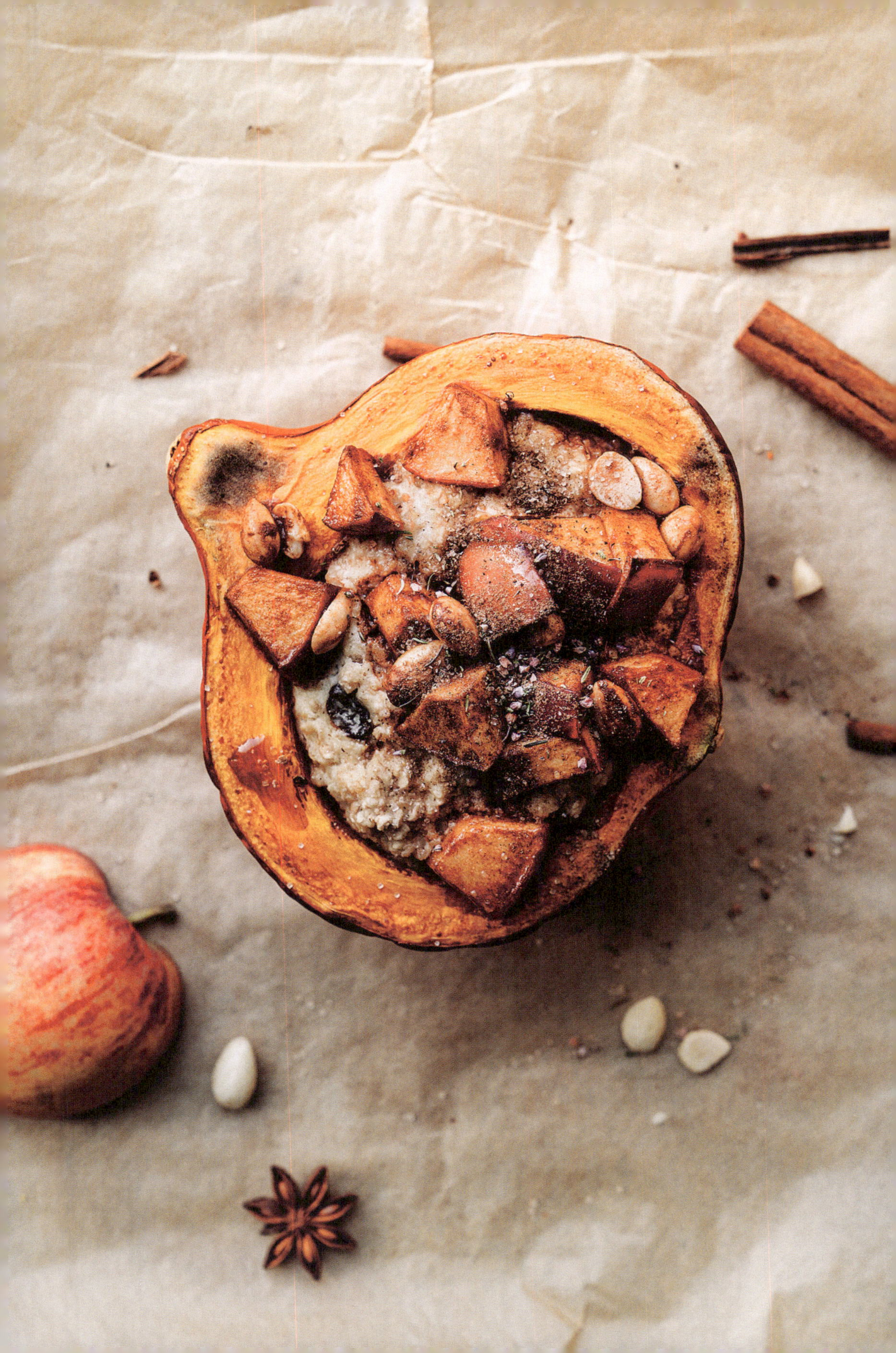

GOOD MOOD SMOOTHIE BOWL

SERVES 1

FOR THE RAWNOLA *(makes 3 portions)*
80 g pitted dates (preferably soft, e.g. Medjool)
30 g thin-rolled porridge oats
30 g + 1 tbsp desiccated coconut
1 pinch of sea salt

FOR THE SMOOTHIE
2 (200 g) frozen bananas
2 tbsp cocoa powder
1 tbsp plant-based protein powder (e.g. pea, rice, soya)
1 tbsp almond butter
2 tsp maple syrup (optional)
75 ml plant-based milk

EXTRAS
Fruit of your choice (e.g. banana, raspberries)
Dark chocolate, chopped

To make the rawnola, blend all the ingredients together (except the 1 tablespoon of desiccated coconut) in a blender. Transfer the mixture to a bowl and add the remaining desiccated coconut. Knead the mixture into a sticky dough, then break it up into crumbs with your fingers.

To make the smoothie, put all the ingredients into a blender and blend until smooth and creamy.

When ready to serve, fill a bowl with the smoothie and top with a portion of rawnola, fruit of your choice and chopped dark chocolate.

· NOTE ·
Rawnola ('raw granola') makes a good alternative to your typical baked granola. It can be both a delicious component of breakfast bowls and a tasty and nutritious snack for in between meals. Rawnola can stay fresh for several weeks if kept in the fridge, although it will rarely last that long.

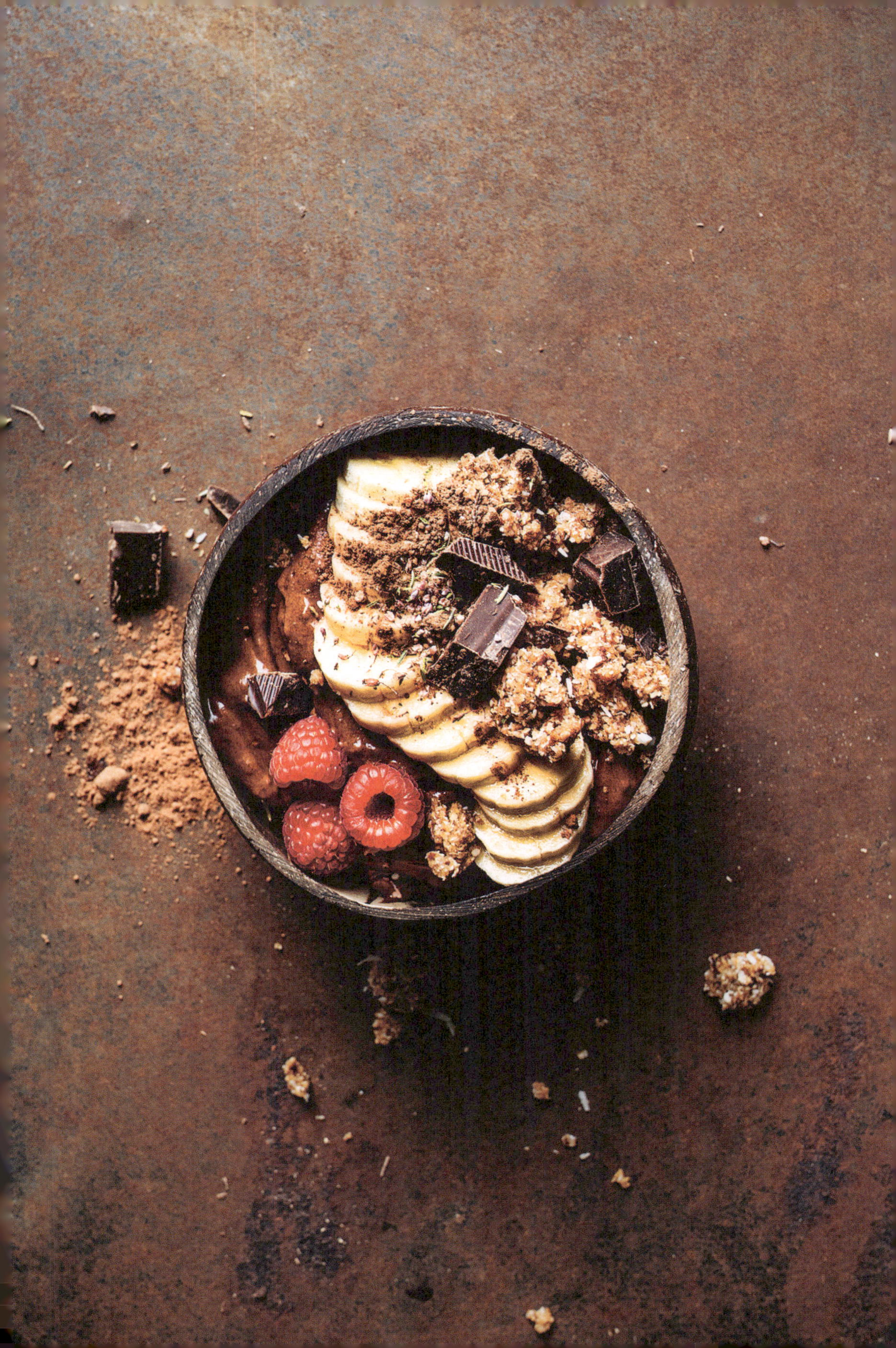

'EAT THE RAINBOW' BREAKFAST PIZZA

MAKES 1

FOR THE BASE

100 g thin-rolled porridge oats
100 g unsweetened apple sauce
30 g desiccated coconut
20 g ground almonds
1 tbsp chia seeds
1 tbsp maple syrup

FOR THE TOPPING

200 g soya quark
Colourful fruit of your choice (e.g. blueberries, strawberries, kiwi)
Toppings of your choice (e.g. desiccated coconut, mint, nut butter)

To make the base, mix all the ingredients in a bowl to form a dough. Transfer the dough to a sheet of baking paper and flatten it with your hands into a disc. If the dough sticks, moisten your hands with a little water. Preheat the oven to 180°C and allow the pizza base to rest in the meantime.

Bake the pizza base for about 20 minutes, until the edges turn a nice golden brown colour. Then remove it from the oven, transfer to a rack and allow to cool completely.

In the meantime, stir the quark until creamy and prepare the fruit for the topping.

Spread the base with quark and then arrange the fruit on top (optionally, by colour). Serve the breakfast pizza with toppings of your choice.

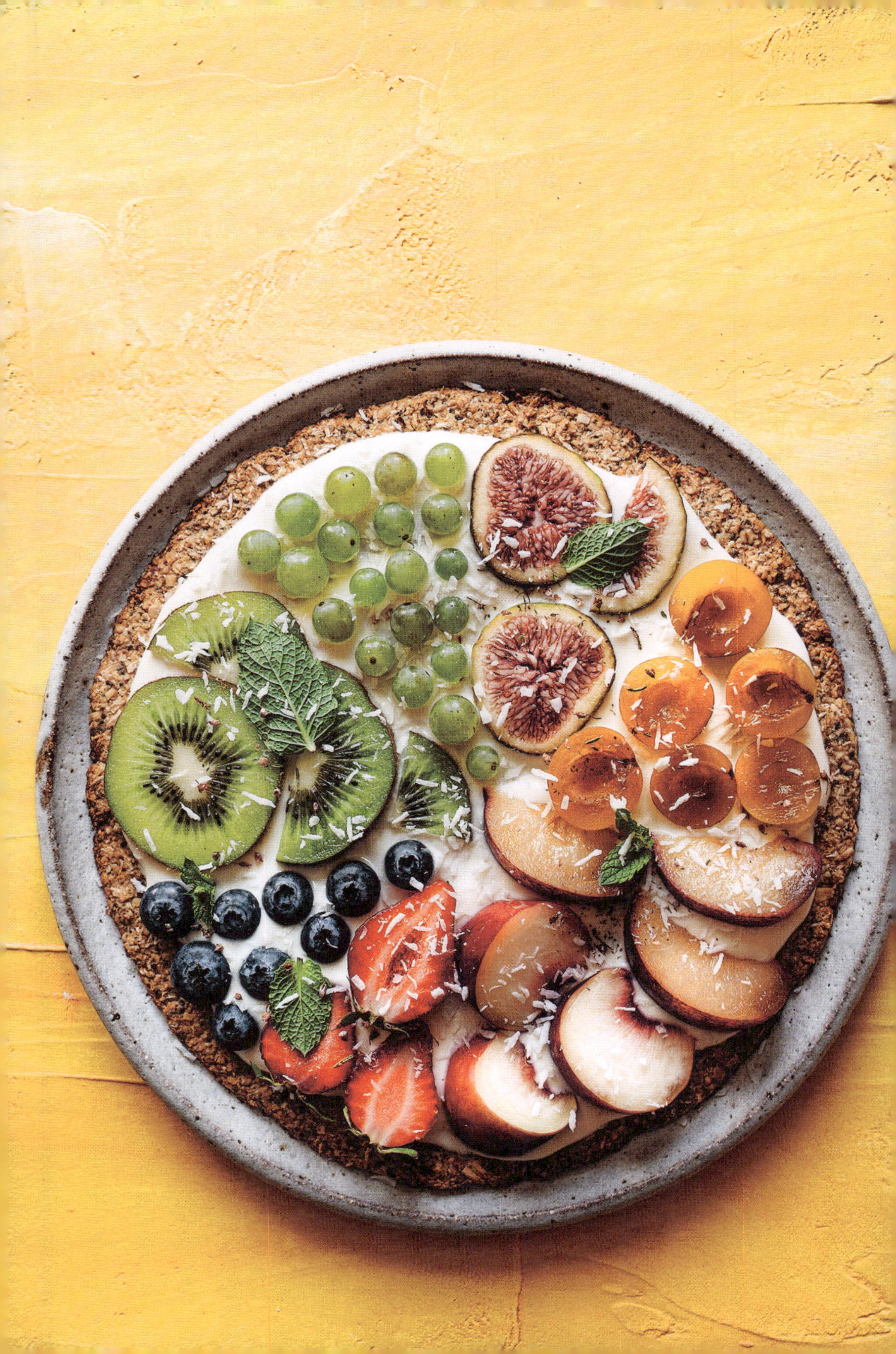

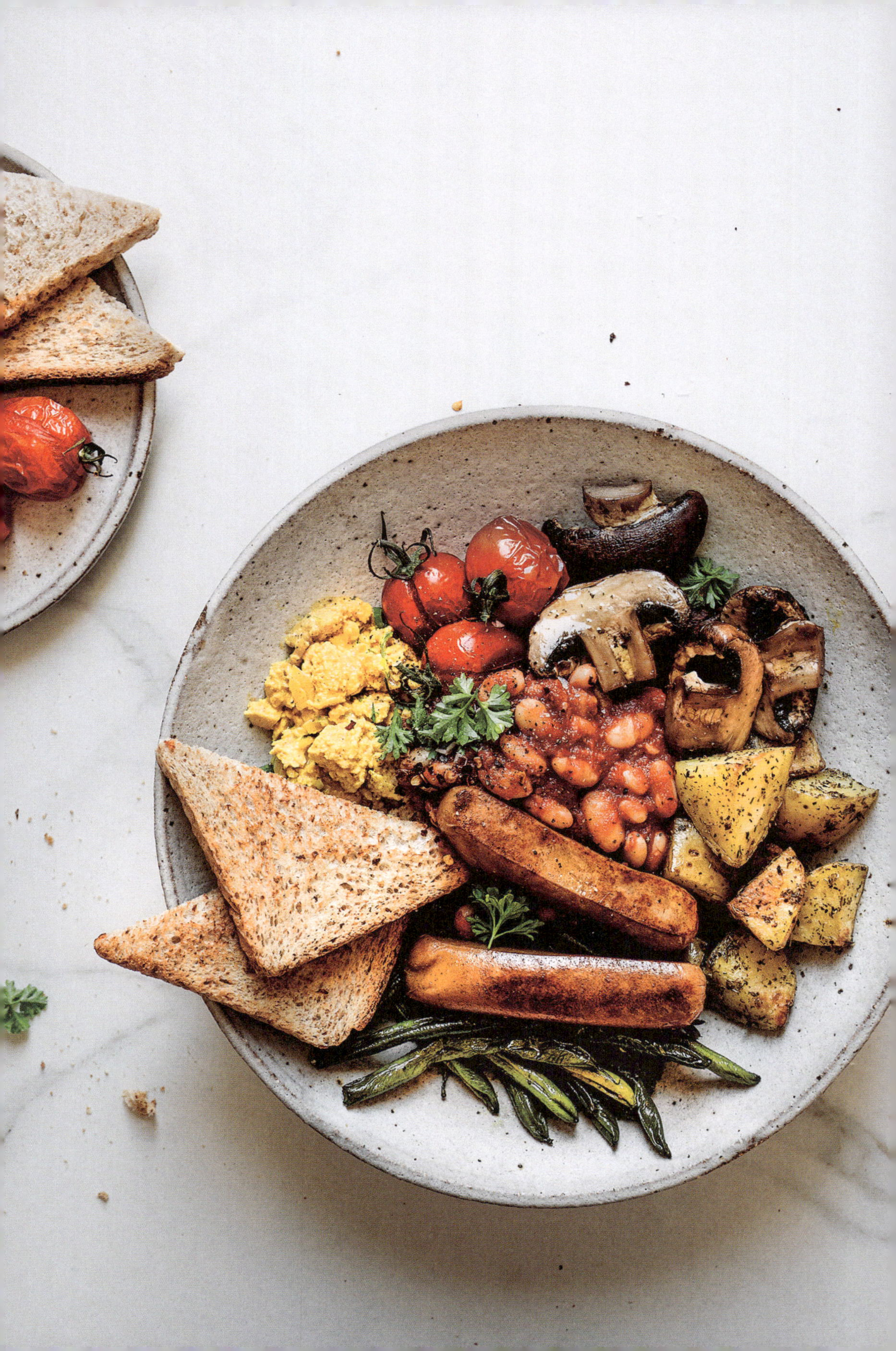

'FULL ENGLISH' BREAKFAST BOWL

SERVES 2

FOR THE BAKED BEANS

250 g cooked haricot beans
400 g tinned chopped tomatoes
1 clove garlic, crushed
1 tbsp agave syrup
2 tsp white wine vinegar
Sea salt, freshly ground pepper, cayenne pepper

FOR THE ROASTED VEGETABLES

2 medium potatoes
2 tbsp olive oil
Sea salt, freshly ground pepper
1 tsp dried Italian herbs
2 handfuls dwarf French beans
8 cherry vine tomatoes
6 chestnut mushrooms

FOR THE SCRAMBLED TOFU

200 g firm tofu
2 tsp rapeseed oil
1 spring onion, sliced
¼ tsp ground turmeric
4 tbsp unsweetened soya yoghurt
½ tsp kala namak (sulphur-rich Indian black salt, available from health food shops)
Sea salt, freshly ground pepper

EXTRAS

4 vegan sausages
Rapeseed oil
2 slices wholemeal bread
Curly parsley, plucked

Preheat the oven to 200°C.

To make the baked beans, place the beans in a sieve, rinse thoroughly under running water and allow to drain. Put the beans into a pan with the remaining ingredients and bring to the boil. Reduce the heat to low and allow to simmer for a few minutes. Season with salt and the spices, cover and set aside.

To make the roasted vegetables, wash the potatoes, quarter them lengthways and cut into finger-thick chunks. Mix them with the oil in a bowl and spread them over a baking tray lined with baking paper (set aside the bowl with the leftover oil). Season with salt and pepper, sprinkle with the herbs and roast for 15 minutes.

In the meantime, wash the green beans, pat dry and trim the stalk tops, then rub them with the oil left over from the potatoes. Wash the tomatoes and clean and halve the mushrooms. After 15 minutes, when the potatoes are half-cooked, add the vegetables to the tray and roast for a further 15 minutes until everything is cooked through.

To make the scrambled tofu, drain the tofu, then place the block in a bowl and crumble it up using your fingers. Heat the oil in a frying pan and fry the tofu for a few minutes. Add the spring onion rings and turmeric and allow the turmeric to toast for 30 seconds while stirring constantly. Remove the pan from the heat, stir in the soya yoghurt and season the scrambled tofu with kala namak, salt and pepper.

Fry the sausages in a frying pan with a little oil and toast the bread. Divide the roasted vegetables, scrambled tofu and a portion of baked beans between two bowls, then add the sausages and wholemeal toast and garnish with fresh parsley.

BANANA BREAD WITH DATES AND TOASTED WALNUTS

MAKES 1 LOAF (25-CM-LONG LOAF TIN)

100 g shelled walnuts
100 g pitted dates
3 (300 g) ripe bananas
150 ml plant-based milk
1 tbsp apple cider vinegar
250 g wholemeal spelt flour
1 tbsp ground cinnamon
8 g baking powder

Preheat the oven to 180°C.

Coarsely chop the walnuts and toast them in a dry non-stick frying pan over a high heat while stirring until fragrant. Transfer to a bowl and set aside. Slice the dates and set aside.

In a bowl, mash the bananas with a fork, then mix with the plant-based milk and vinegar until smooth. In a large bowl, mix the flour with the cinnamon, baking powder and toasted walnuts. Add the mashed banana mixture and mix until combined. Finally, gently mix in the dates.

Spoon the mixture into a loaf tin lined with baking paper and bake for about 40 minutes (test with a bamboo skewer). Remove the banana bread from the oven, lift it out of the tin and allow it to cool before slicing.

· NOTE ·

This bread will stay fresh for a week if stored in the fridge. It is also suitable for freezing, preferably cut into slices.

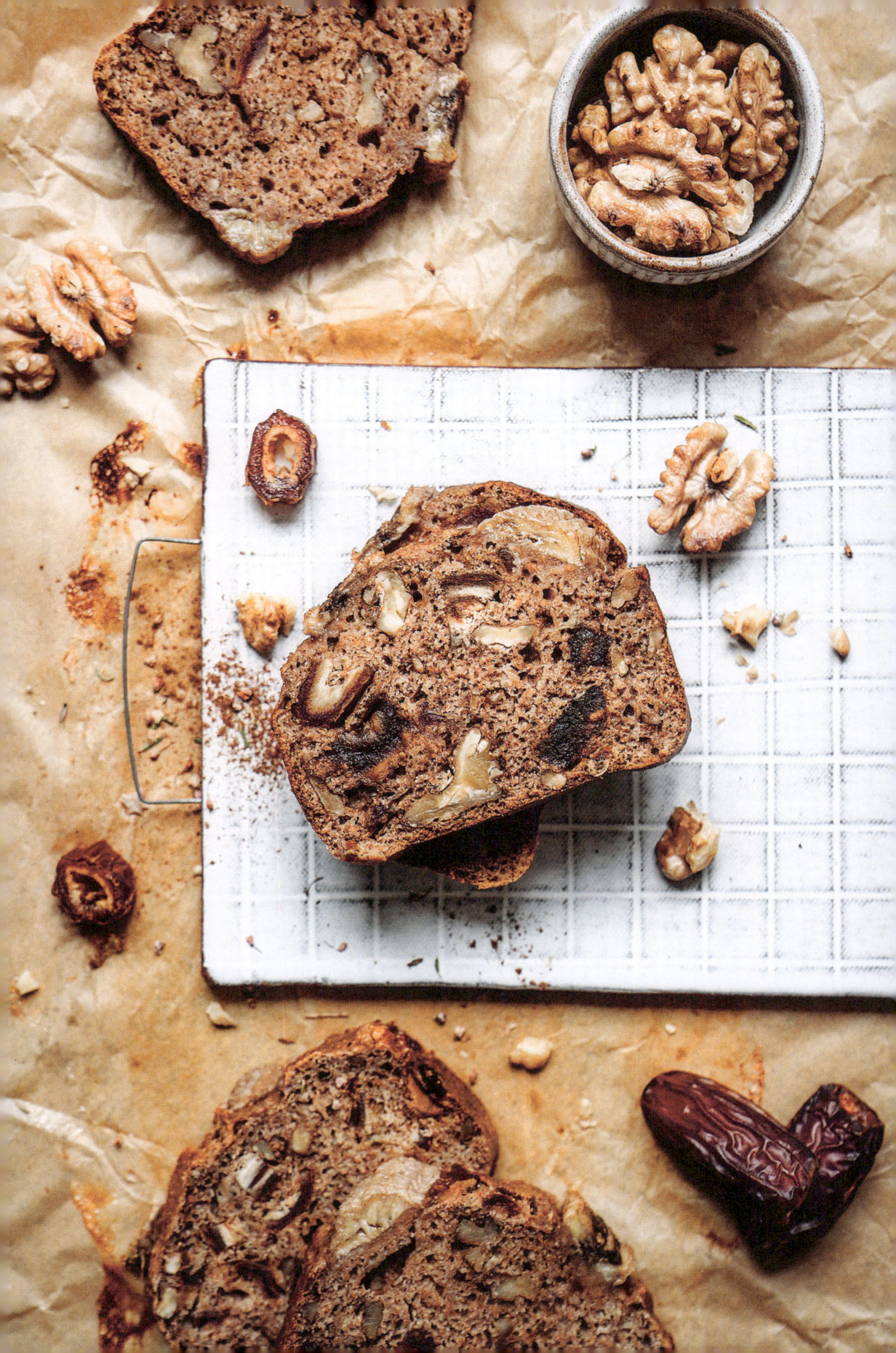

WHOLESOME SEED & NUT BREAD

MAKES 1 LOAF (25-CM-LONG LOAF TIN)

- 130 g thin-rolled porridge oats
- 80 g linseed
- 80 g sunflower seeds
- 80 g pumpkin seeds
- 80 g nuts of your choice (e.g. pecans, walnuts, hazelnuts), coarsely chopped
- 4 tbsp psyllium husks
- 3 tbsp hemp seeds (or substitute with sesame seeds)
- 2 tbsp chia seeds
- 1 tsp sea salt
- 3 tbsp coconut oil, melted
- 2 tbsp sugar (or substitute with maple syrup)
- 1 tbsp balsamic vinegar

Mix all the dry ingredients together in a large bowl. In another bowl, mix the coconut oil, sugar and vinegar with 350 ml of warm water, then add to the dry ingredients and mix until combined. Line a loaf tin with baking paper and add the dough one portion at a time, pressing down firmly each time, until filled. Cover the tin and rest the dough in the fridge for at least 4 hours (preferably overnight) so the mixture can fully absorb the liquid.

Preheat the oven to 180°C. Bake the bread for 30 minutes, then hold the baking paper and lift it out of the tin (do this very carefully as it will be very hot). Turn the loaf over onto the oven rack (without the tin) and bake for a further 30 minutes. Remove the bread from the oven and leave it to cool completely before slicing.

• NOTE •

This bread will stay fresh for a week if stored in the fridge. It is also suitable for freezing, preferably cut into slices.

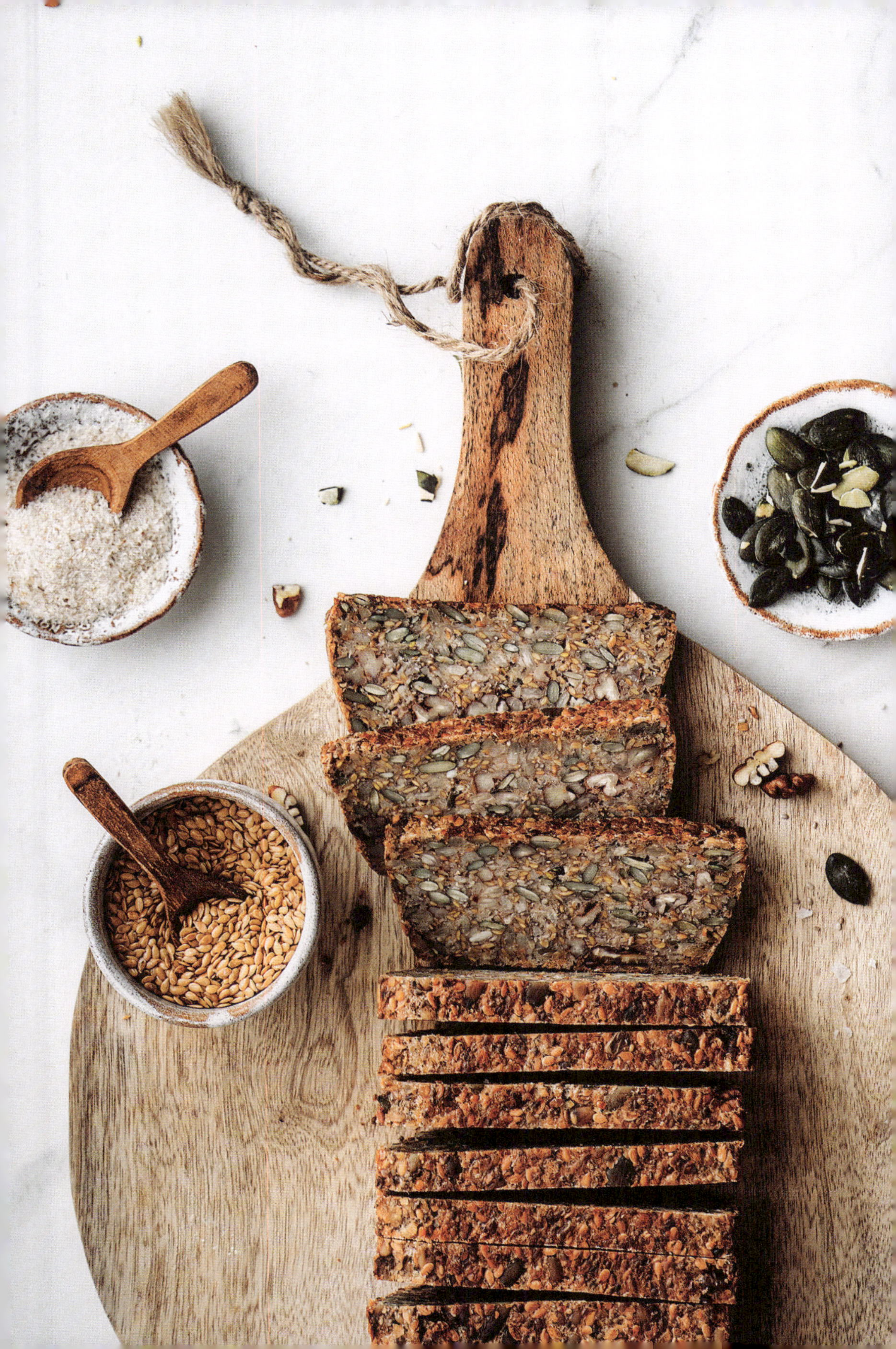

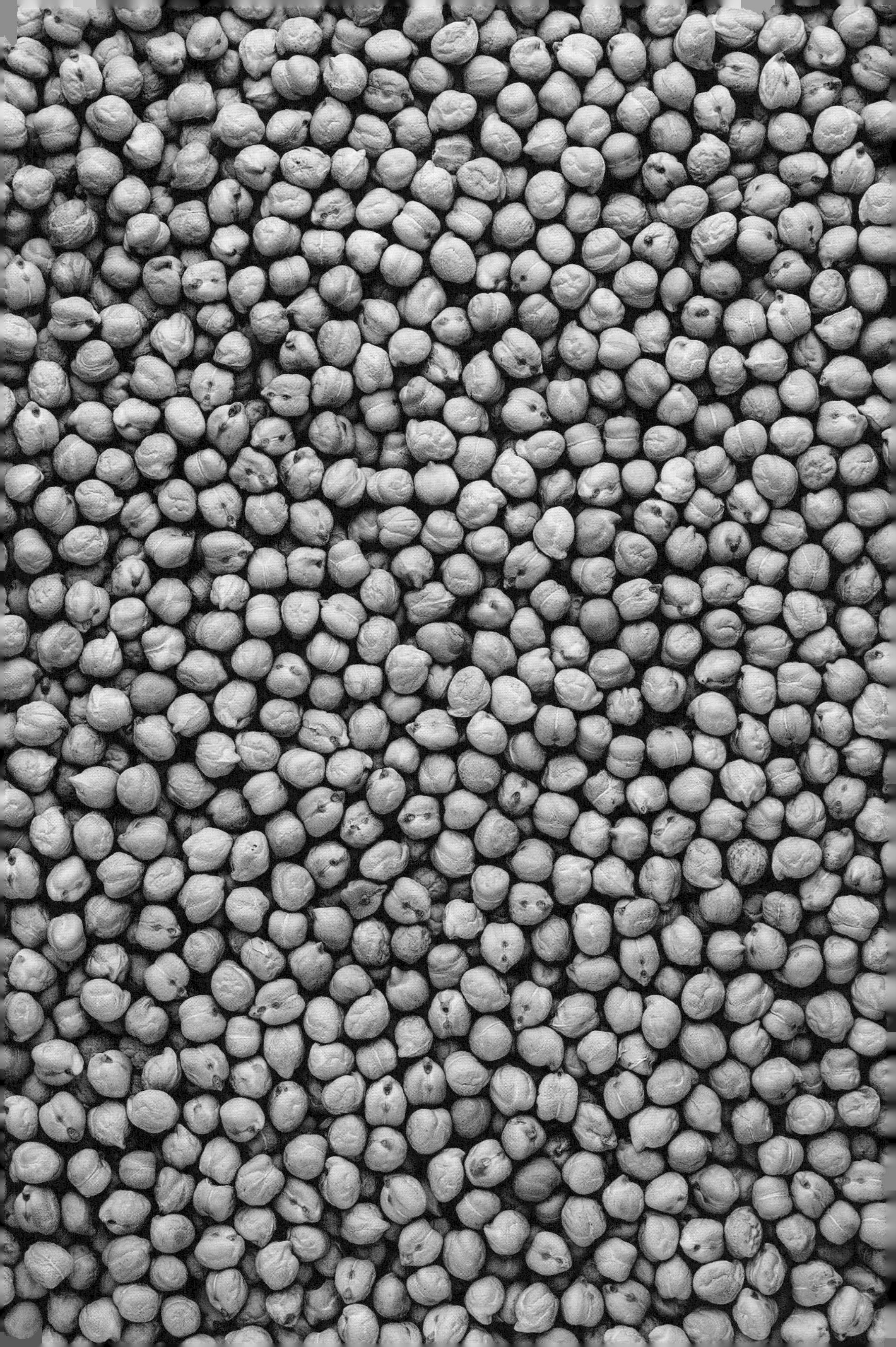

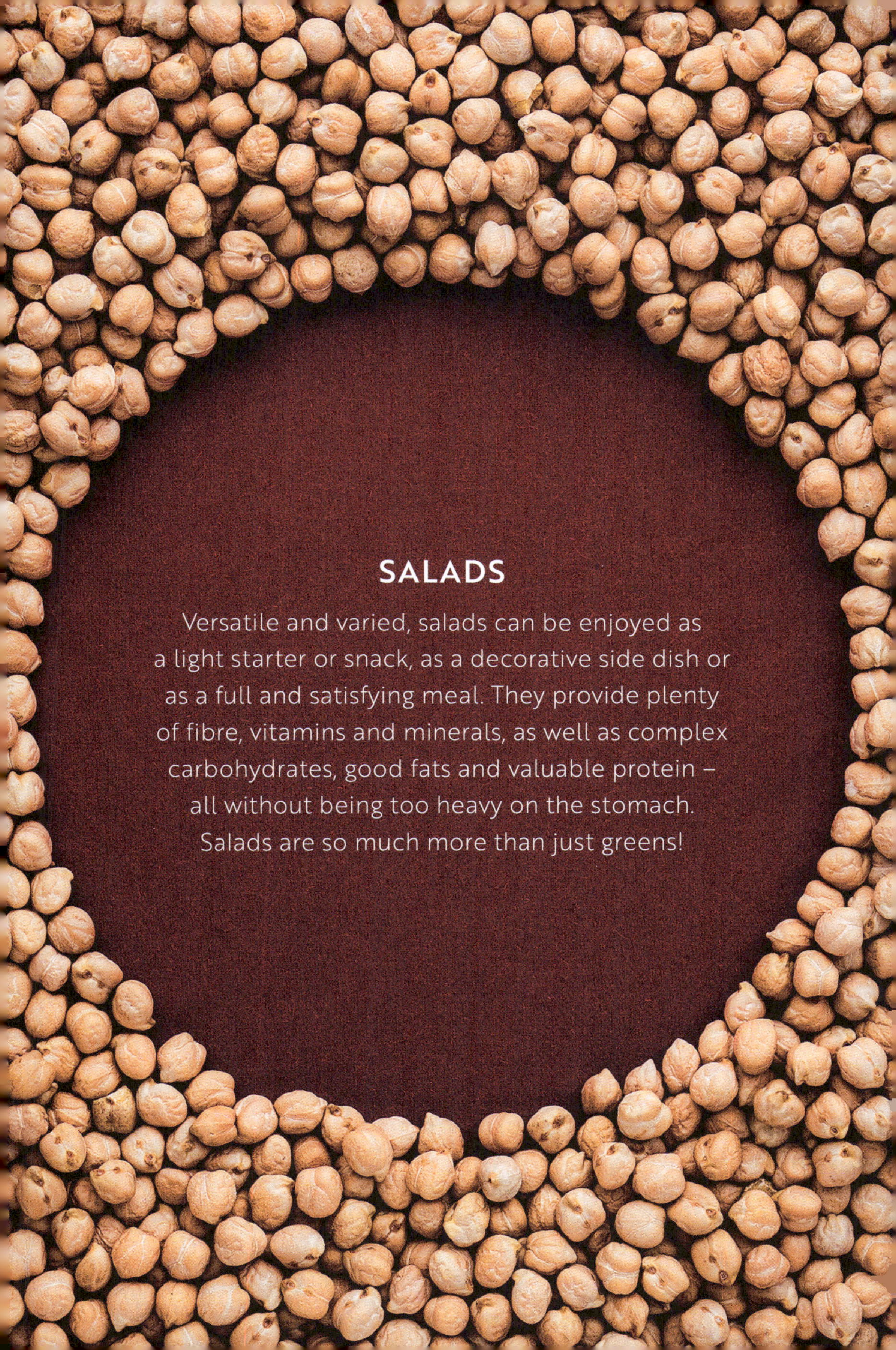

SALADS

Versatile and varied, salads can be enjoyed as a light starter or snack, as a decorative side dish or as a full and satisfying meal. They provide plenty of fibre, vitamins and minerals, as well as complex carbohydrates, good fats and valuable protein – all without being too heavy on the stomach. Salads are so much more than just greens!

COLOURFUL CONFETTI SALAD

SERVES 6

FOR THE SALAD

250 g couscous
4 spring onions
1 red pepper
1 yellow pepper
1 organic cucumber
250 g cooked chickpeas
1 tin sweetcorn (285 g drained weight)

FOR THE DRESSING

3 tbsp olive oil
2 tbsp tomato purée
2 tbsp rice vinegar
2 tbsp soy sauce
2 tbsp freshly squeezed lemon juice
1 tbsp red curry paste (shop-bought or homemade, see page 76)
1 tsp sweet paprika
1 tsp ground cumin
1 tsp ground coriander

EXTRAS

½ bunch parsley, chopped
Sea salt, freshly ground pepper

To make the salad, bring 250 ml of salted water to the boil in a pan. Stir in the couscous, then remove from the heat, cover and allow to stand for 10 minutes.

In the meantime, wash and thinly slice the spring onions. Wash and halve the peppers, remove the seeds and ribs and dice. Wash and finely dice the cucumber. Place the chickpeas and sweetcorn in a sieve, rinse thoroughly under running water and allow to drain. Mix everything together in a large salad bowl.

To make the dressing, mix all the ingredients together in a small bowl.

Mix the couscous with the dressing, then add the dressed couscous to the salad vegetables and toss well. Finally, gently mix the parsley into the salad and season with salt and pepper. Add more seasonings if necessary.

• NOTE •

This confetti salad will taste especially good if made the evening before and allowed to stand overnight.

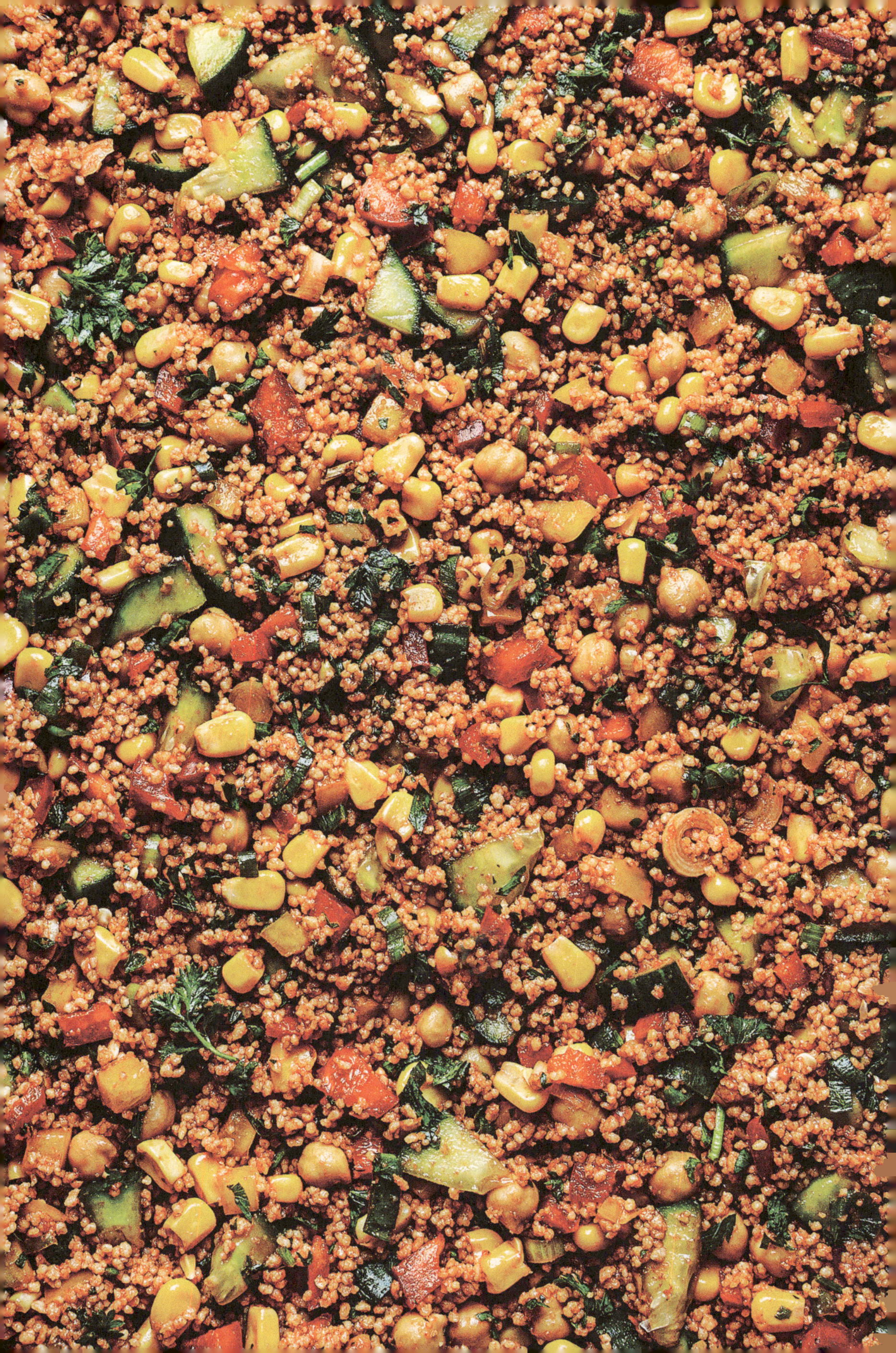

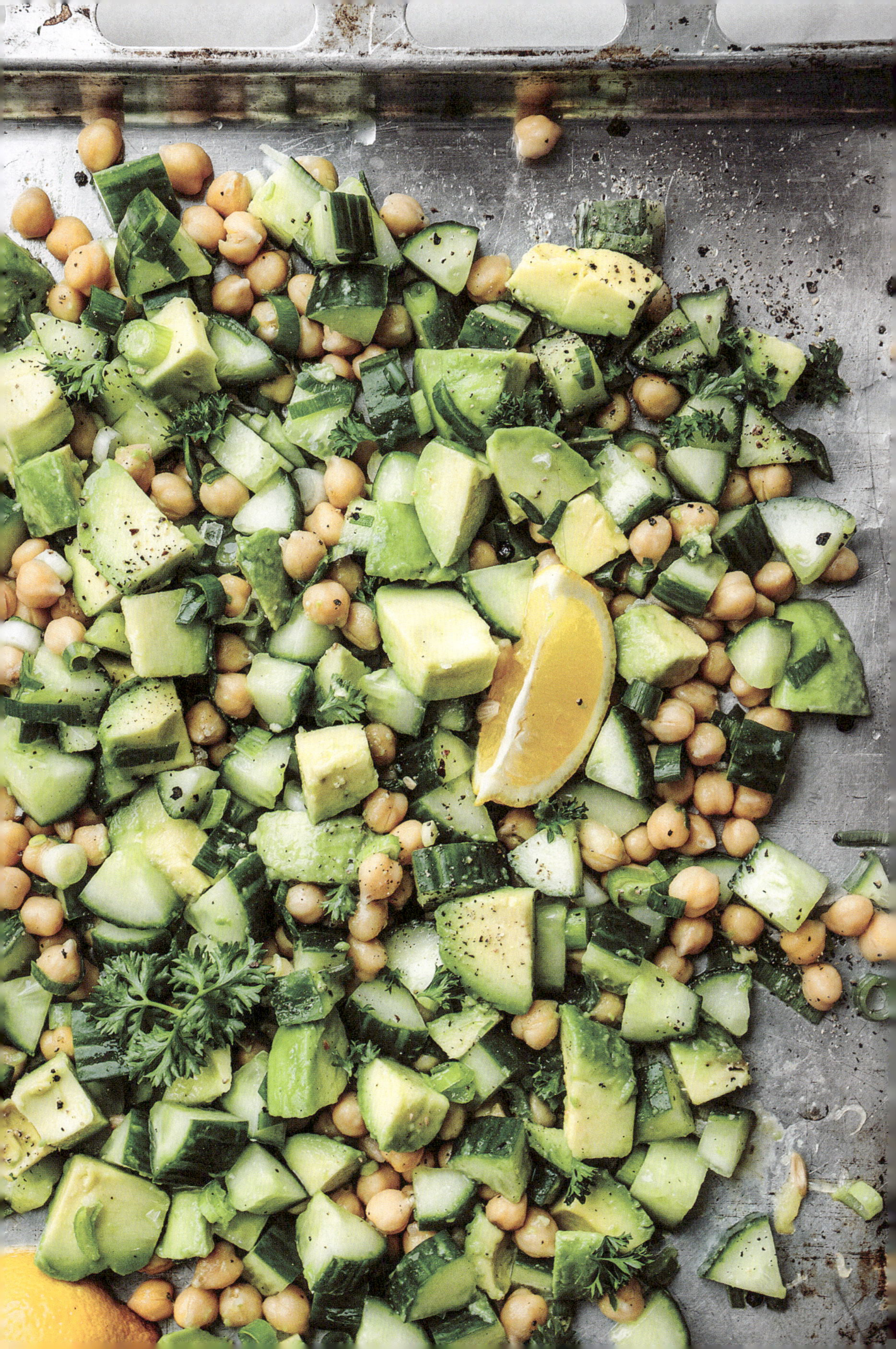

AVOCADO & CHICKPEA SALAD

SERVES 4

250 g cooked chickpeas
1 organic cucumber
3 spring onions
2 avocados
Juice of 1 lemon
Sea salt, freshly ground pepper

Place the chickpeas in a sieve, rinse thoroughly under running water and allow to drain. Wash and finely dice the cucumber. Trim, wash and thinly slice the spring onions. Halve the avocados, remove the stone and score the flesh crossways. Using a spoon, scoop out the flesh and place it in a bowl together with the chickpeas, diced cucumber and spring onions. Drizzle with a little lemon juice and mix carefully. Season with salt and a plenty of pepper. Add more lemon juice if necessary.

• NOTE •

This avocado and chickpea salad tastes best when freshly prepared. However, the lemon juice also allows it to be made in advance and retain its bright green colour.

GREEK SALAD WITH TOFU FETA

SERVES 4

FOR THE TOFU FETA

200 g firm tofu
3 tbsp olive oil
1 tbsp white wine vinegar
3 cloves garlic, crushed
1 tbsp chopped parsley
1 tbsp chopped basil
1 tbsp dried oregano
1 tsp dried thyme
1 tsp sea salt
Freshly ground pepper

FOR THE SALAD

250 g cherry vine tomatoes
1 organic cucumber
1 red onion
80 g pitted black olives from a jar

FOR THE DRESSING

3 tbsp olive oil
2 tbsp white wine vinegar
1 tsp dried oregano
1 tbsp freshly squeezed lemon juice
Sea salt, freshly ground pepper

To make the tofu feta, drain the tofu the day before and cut it into finger-thick slices. Place the slices between sheets of kitchen paper and squeeze out the remaining liquid, then cut them into uniform cubes. Mix all the remaining ingredients for the tofu feta in a large screw-top jar. Then add the tofu cubes, close the jar and shake until the tofu cubes are completely coated in the marinade. Marinate in the fridge for 24 hours (or longer if desired).

To make the salad, wash and halve the tomatoes. Wash and quarter the cucumber lengthways, then cut into small pieces. Peel and thinly slice the onion. Drain the olives in a sieve. Mix everything together in a large salad bowl.

To make the dressing, mix all the ingredients together in a small bowl.

When ready to serve, drizzle the dressing over the salad and toss well. Finally, remove the tofu feta cubes from the marinade and gently mix them into the salad.

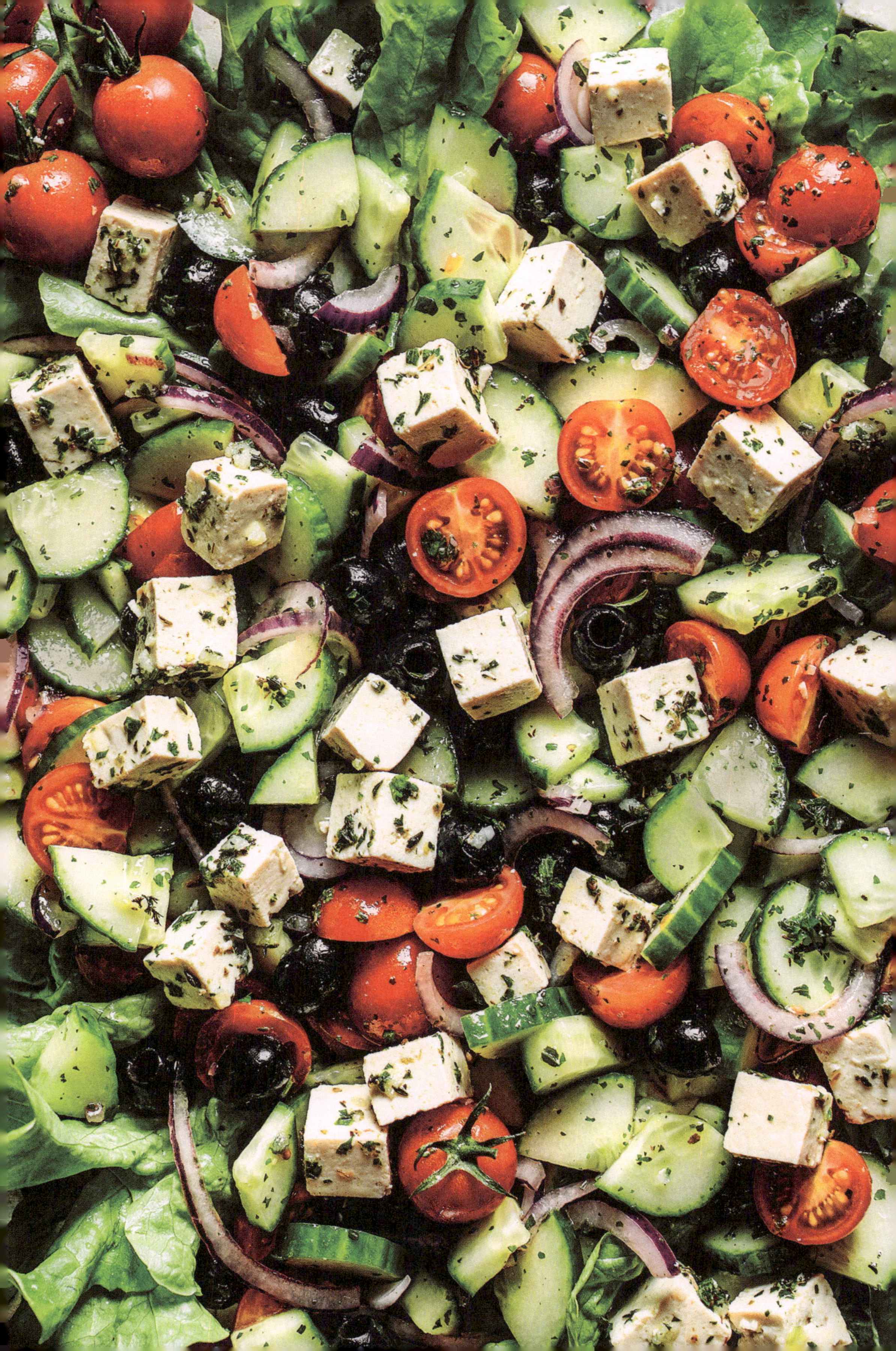

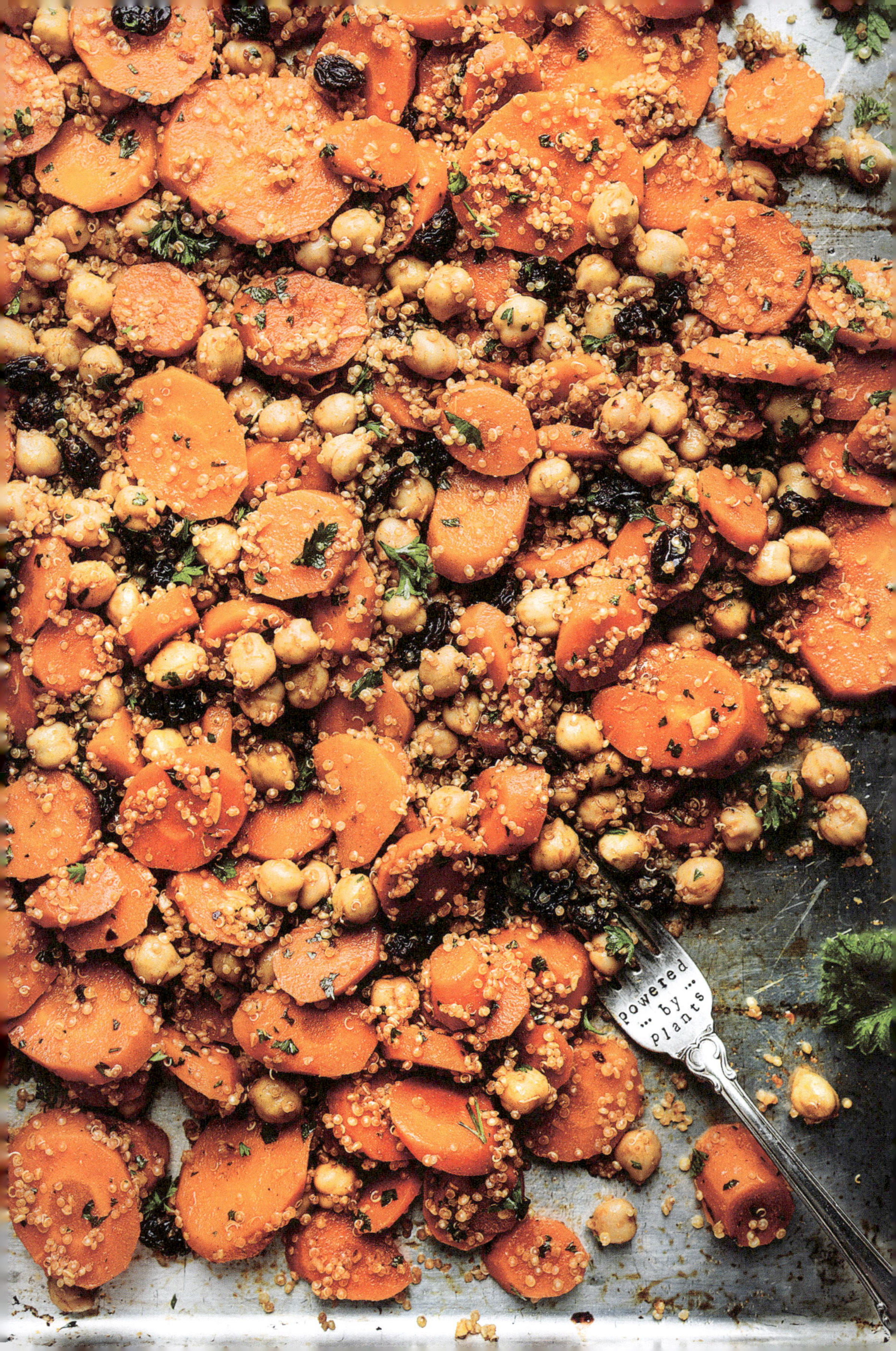
powered
... by ...
plants

MOROCCAN CARROT SALAD

SERVES 4

125 g quinoa
500 g carrots (peeled and trimmed before weighing)
250 g cooked chickpeas
4 cloves garlic
2 tbsp olive oil
1 tsp ground cumin
1 tsp sweet paprika
1 tsp ground cinnamon
60 g raisins
3 tbsp freshly squeezed lemon juice
Sea salt, cayenne pepper
½ bunch parsley, chopped

Cook the quinoa according to the packet instructions and set aside.

Bring salted water to the boil in a pan. Cut the peeled carrots slightly on a diagonal into 5-mm-thick slices. Cook them in salted water until still firm to the bite (not until soft), then drain in a sieve and transfer to a bowl.

Place the chickpeas in a sieve, rinse thoroughly under running water and allow to drain. Peel and finely chop the garlic.

Gently heat the oil in a frying pan. Add the garlic and spices and sauté for 1–2 minutes while stirring constantly. Then add the quinoa, carrots, chickpeas, raisins and lemon juice and mix everything together. Season with salt and cayenne pepper and gently mix in the parsley at the end.

• NOTE •
This carrot salad can be served either warm or cold.

ASIAN-STYLE COLESLAW WITH A SESAME AND GINGER DRESSING

SERVES 4

FOR THE COLESLAW

350 g red cabbage
150 g white cabbage
3 spring onions
2 carrots
200 g mangetout
200 g frozen shelled edamame (available at Oriental supermarkets), thawed
Juice of 1 lime

FOR THE SESAME AND GINGER DRESSING

1 clove garlic, crushed
1 tbsp freshly grated ginger
5 tbsp soy sauce
2 tbsp olive oil
2 tbsp rice vinegar
1 tbsp agave syrup
1 tsp chilli flakes
2 tbsp sesame seeds

EXTRAS

80 g roasted and salted peanuts, chopped
1 handful coriander leaves, picked

To make the coleslaw, clean and trim both types of cabbage and shred them using a mandoline or knife. Wash, trim and slice the spring onions, carrots and mangetout and cut into very thin strips. Mix everything together with the edamame in a large bowl and drizzle with the lime juice.

To make the dressing, mix all the ingredients together in a small bowl.

When ready to serve, drizzle the dressing over the salad and toss well. Scatter the chopped peanuts and coriander over the coleslaw and serve.

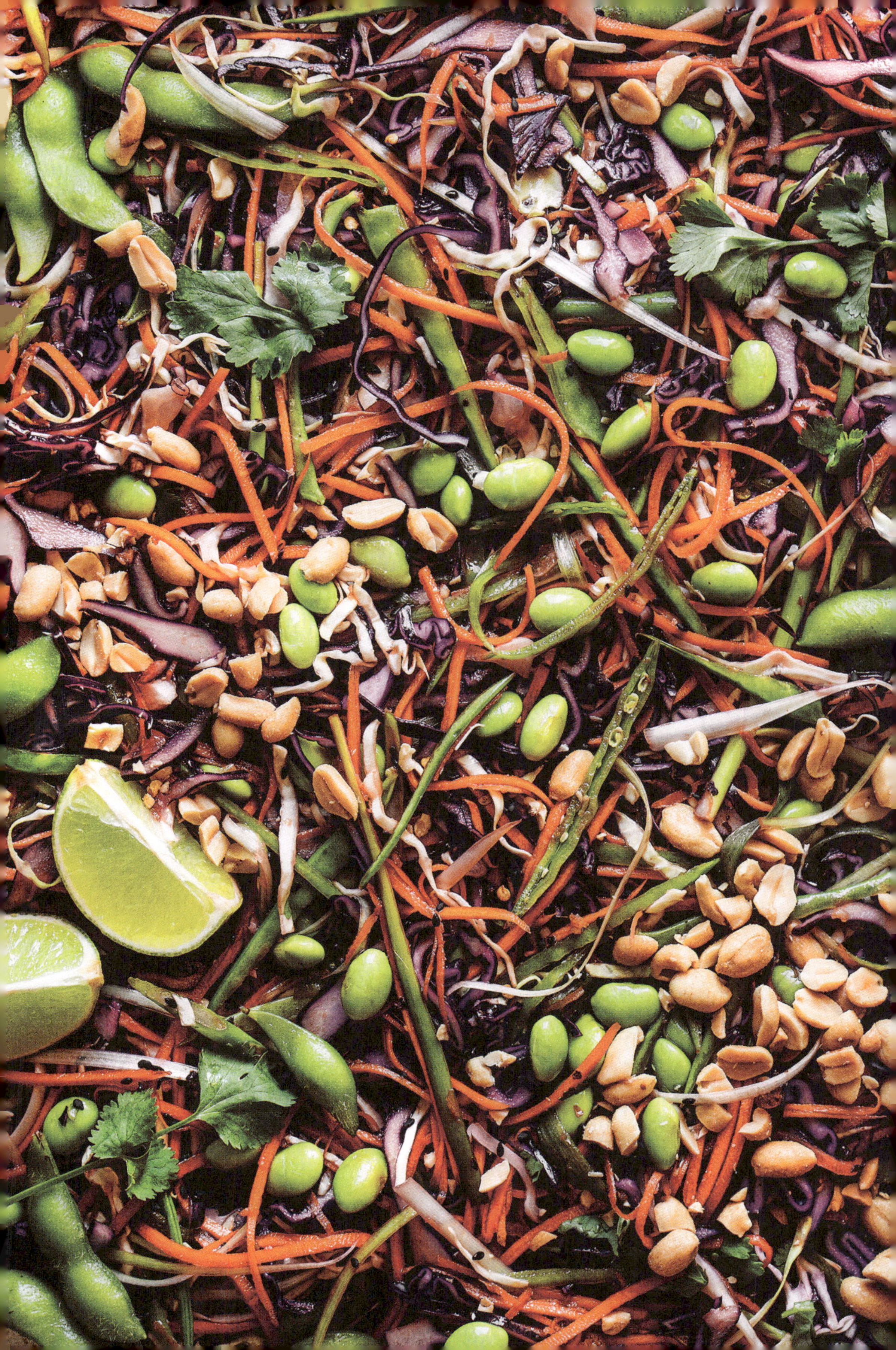

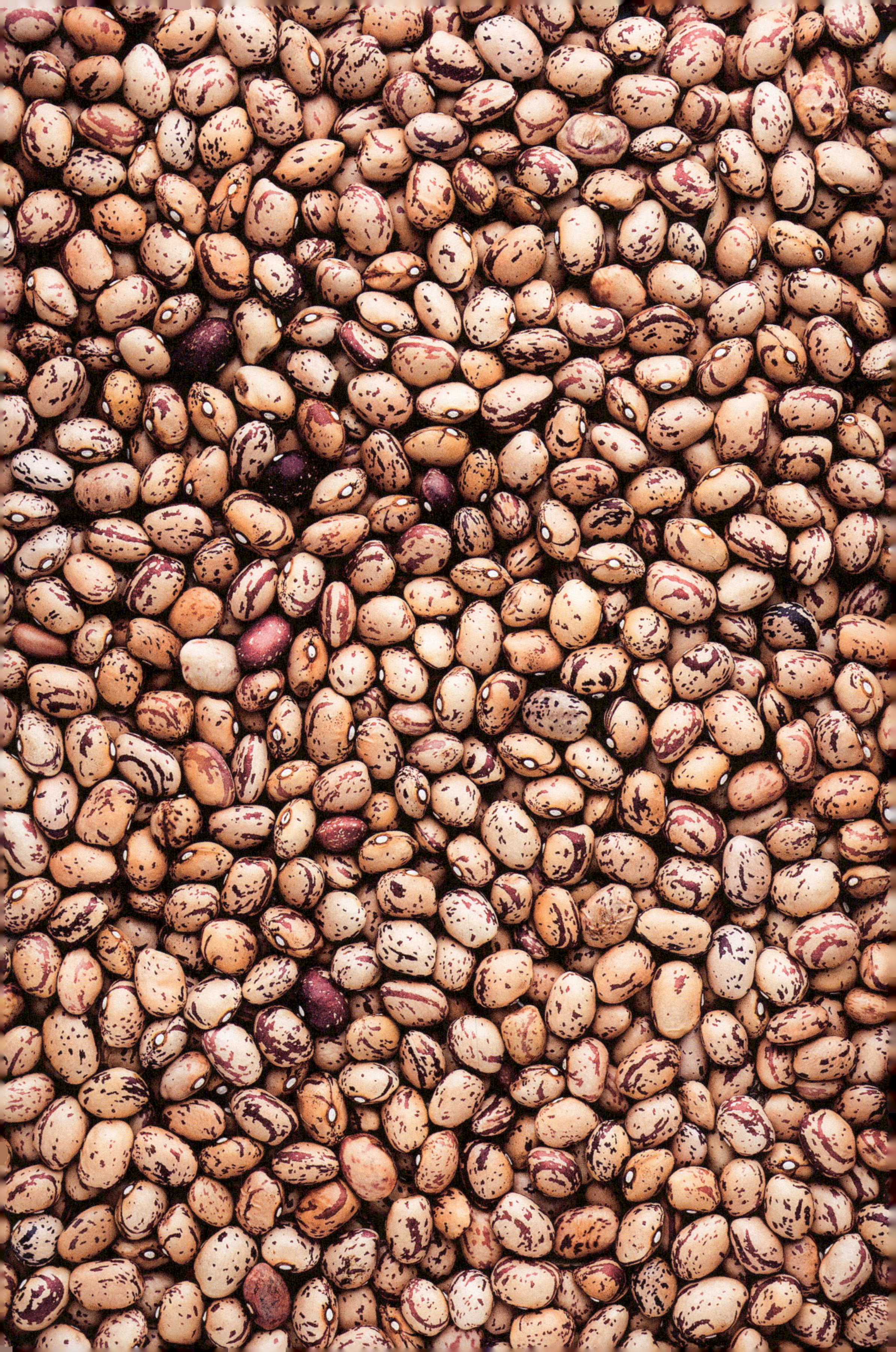

BOWLS

Colourful bowls packed full of healthy ingredients are a feast for both the eyes and the palate. Healthy food has never been so visually appealing, creative and delicious. This chapter contains the recipes for five different bowls to inspire your own creations. Whether to follow the whole recipes or just make use of some of their components is entirely up to you. Happy bowling.

BURRITO BOWL

FOR 2 BOWLS

FOR THE TOMATO SALSA

2 vine tomatoes
½ red onion
1 clove garlic
½ red pepper
1–2 tbsp finely chopped coriander
Juice of ½ lime
Sea salt, freshly ground pepper

FOR THE BOWL

150 g basmati rice
1 red pepper
1 yellow pepper
1 ear fresh sweetcorn
Rapeseed oil
250 g cooked black beans
1 head Cos lettuce
1 avocado

EXTRAS

Toppings of your choice (e.g. lime, coriander, chilli flakes)
Chipotle sauce (see page 120, or substitute with the sauce of your choice)

To make the tomato salsa, wash and halve the tomatoes, then cut off the stem end, de-seed and cut into small dice. Peel the onion and garlic, wash the chilli peppers and cut everything into very small dice. Put everything into a bowl, add the coriander and mix the ingredients together. Drizzle with lime juice, season with salt and pepper and set aside.

For the bowl, cook the rice according to the packet instructions and set aside.

Wash and halve the peppers, remove the seeds and membranes and cut into strips. Using a sharp knife, slice the sweetcorn kernels from the cob. Heat a little oil in a non-stick frying pan, add the pepper strips, sauté and transfer to a container. Then do the same with the sweetcorn kernels.

Place the beans in a sieve, rinse thoroughly under running water and allow to drain. Wash and trim the lettuce and cut the leaves into strips.

When ready to serve, divide the rice, salsa, fried vegetables, beans and lettuce between two bowls. Halve the avocado, remove the stone and score the flesh in the centre. Using a spoon, scoop out the flesh and divide it between the bowls. Serve the burrito bowls with toppings of your choice and chipotle sauce.

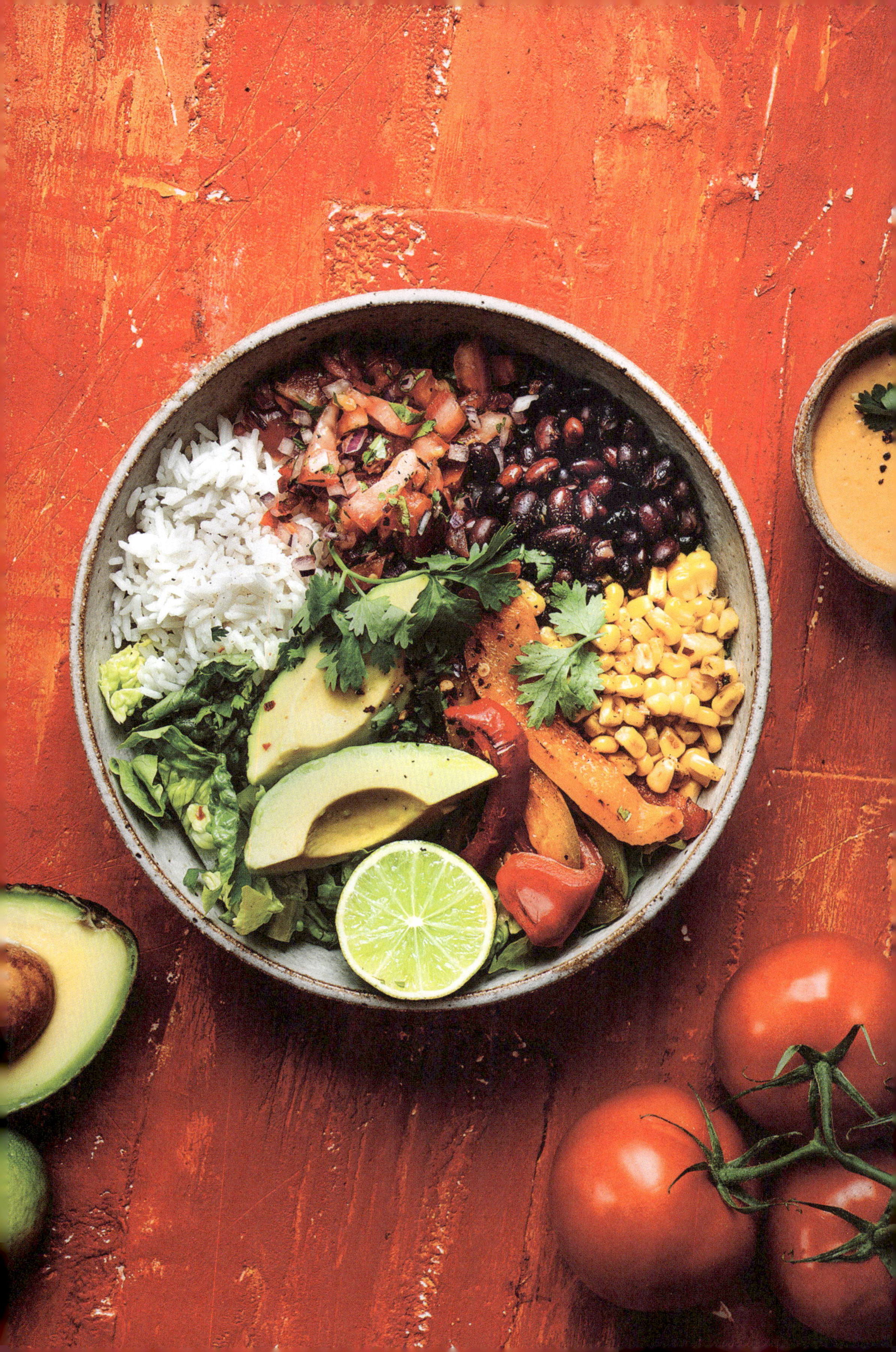

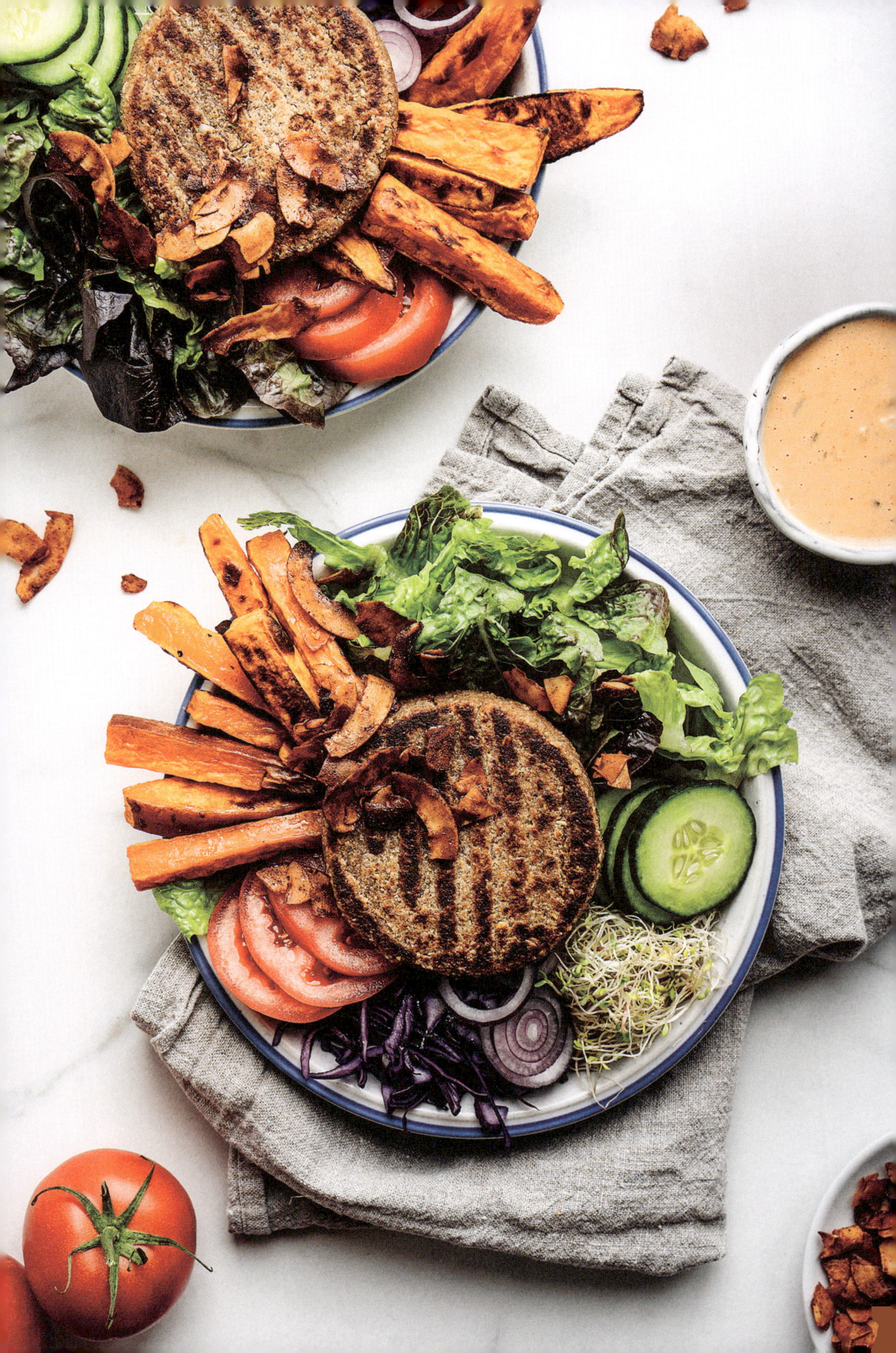

BURGER BOWL

FOR 2 BOWLS

FOR THE SWEET POTATO CHIPS

1 large (500 g) sweet potato
1 tbsp olive oil
Sea salt

FOR THE GREEN SPELT BURGERS

50 g sunflower seeds
100 g green spelt groats
1 shallot
2 cloves garlic
Rapeseed oil
200 ml hot vegetable stock
2–3 tbsp wholemeal spelt flour
1 tbsp yeast flakes
1 dash liquid smoke
Sea salt, freshly ground pepper

FOR THE BOWL

1 head Cos lettuce
1 vine tomato
½ organic cucumber
½ small red onion
1 handful red cabbage
1 handful sprouts of your choice

EXTRAS

Coconut bacon (see page 116, optional)
Burger sauce (see page 120; substitute with the sauce of your choice)

Preheat the oven to 220°C.

To make the chips, wash the sweet potato and cut it into chip-sized batons. Put them into a bowl and mix with the oil and a little salt. Spread the chips over a baking tray lined with baking paper and bake for 25–30 minutes (depending on size), turning them over after 15 minutes.

In the meantime, make the spelt burgers. Finely grind the sunflower seeds in a blender, mix with the green spelt groats and set aside. Peel and finely chop the shallot and garlic. Heat 1 teaspoon of oil in a pan and sauté the shallot and garlic. Add the green spelt mixture, followed by the hot vegetable stock and cook for 1–2 minutes, until considerably thickened. Turn off the heat. Then stir in the flour, yeast flakes and a dash of liquid smoke. Season with salt and pepper and allow the pan to stand on the still-warm hob for 15 minutes.

In the meantime, wash and trim the ingredients for the bowl, peel the onion and cut everything into bite-sized pieces.

Divide the warm green spelt mixture in half and shape two burgers. Heat 1 tablespoon of oil in a frying pan and fry the burgers over high heat for 3–5 minutes on each side, until golden brown.

When ready to serve, divide the sweet potato chips, vegetables, lettuce and sprouts between two bowls and place a burger in the middle of each. Top the burgers with coconut bacon and burger sauce and serve.

SAFARI BOWL

FOR 2 BOWLS

FOR THE SWEET POTATO

1 medium (300 g) sweet potato
1 tbsp agave syrup
1 tsp coconut oil, melted
1 tsp ground cumin
½ tsp ground turmeric
1 tsp ground cinnamon
½ tsp sea salt
1 pinch of cayenne pepper

FOR THE PLANTAINS

2 ripe plantains (yellow to black)
2 tsp coconut oil, melted
1 pinch of sea salt

FOR THE BOWL

100 g couscous
250 g cooked pinto beans (substitute with kidney beans or black-eyed beans)
2 handfuls loose-leaf lettuce, cleaned
2 handfuls roasted and salted peanuts

EXTRAS

Toppings of your choice (e.g. lime, coriander, chilli flakes)
Peanut dip (see recipe on page 119)

Preheat the oven to 220°C.

Peel and cut the sweet potato into thumb-thick chunks. In a large bowl, mix the agave syrup with the coconut oil and spices. Add the sweet potato chunks and coat well. Spread the sweet potato over a baking tray lined with baking paper and bake for 15 minutes.

In the meantime, peel the plantains and cut them slightly on a diagonal into 1.5-cm-thick slices. Transfer to a bowl and mix with the coconut oil and salt. After 15 minutes, when the sweet potato is half-cooked, turn the pieces over and then add the plantain pieces to the tray. Bake for a further 15 minutes, until the plantains are lightly caramelised and the sweet potato is cooked through (watch closely to keep from burning).

In the meantime, bring 150 ml of water to the boil in a small pan. Stir in the couscous, then turn off the heat, cover and allow to stand on the still-warm hob for 15 minutes. Place the beans in a sieve, rinse thoroughly under running water and allow to drain.

When ready to serve, divide the couscous, beans, lettuce, peanuts, sweet potato and plantains between two bowls and serve with toppings of your choice. Accompany with the peanut dip.

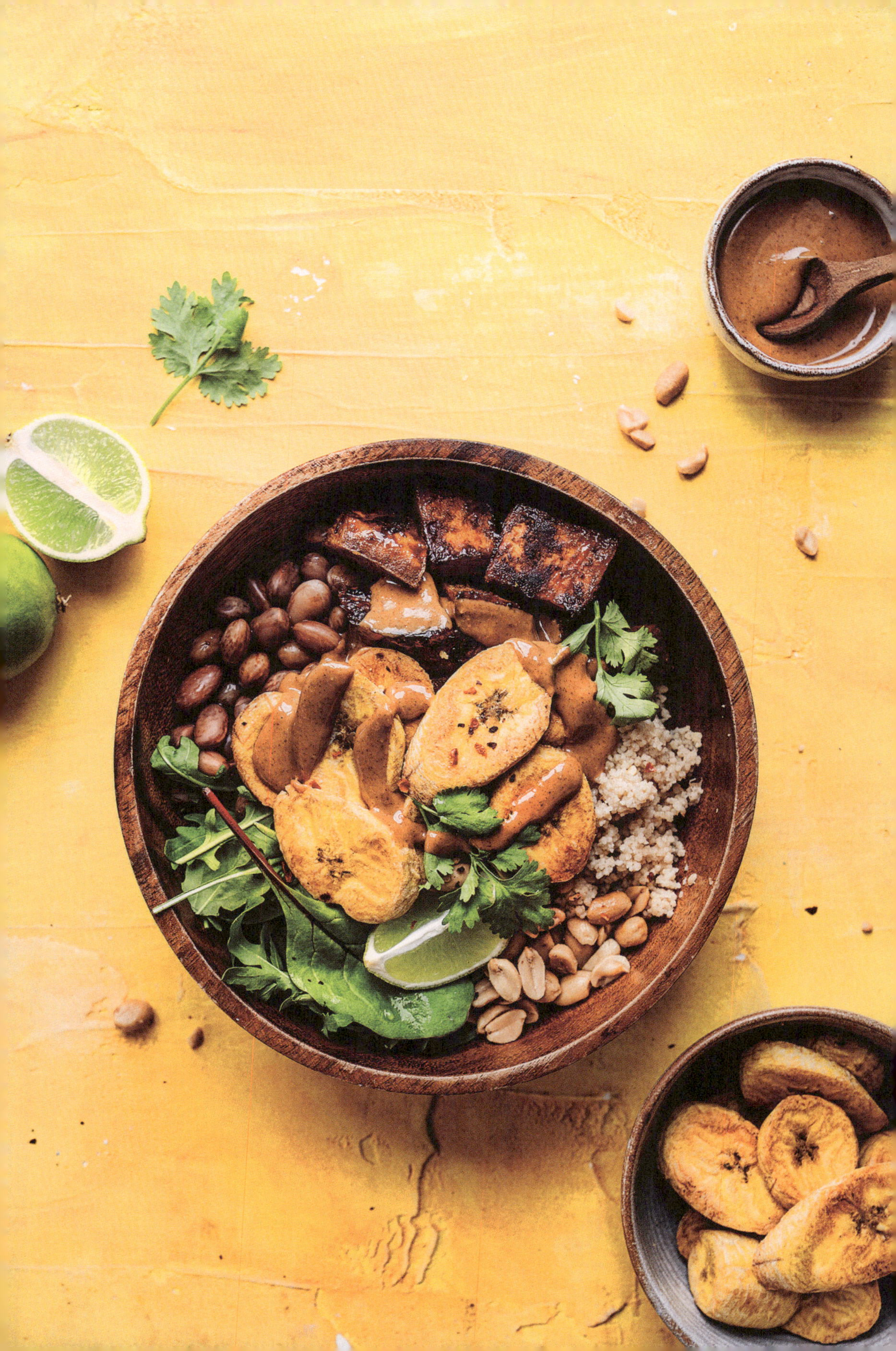

SUSHI BOWL

FOR 2 BOWLS

FOR THE RICE

150 g jasmine rice
1 tbsp rice vinegar
1 tsp agave syrup
Sea salt

FOR THE FRIED TOFU CUBES

200 g firm tofu
1–2 tbsp cornflour
Rapeseed oil

FOR THE BOWL

⅓ organic cucumber
1 carrot
1 spring onion
1 vine tomato
1 handful red cabbage
1 dash rice vinegar
1 avocado
150 g frozen shelled edamame (available at Oriental supermarkets), thawed
100 g frozen wakame salad (available from well-stocked Oriental supermarkets, optional), thawed
2 tbsp pickled sushi ginger (available from Oriental supermarkets)

EXTRAS

Toppings of your choice (e.g. sesame seeds, chilli flakes, lime)
Soy sauce

Cook the rice according to the packet instructions. Then mix in the vinegar, agave syrup and a little salt, cover and set aside.

To make the fried tofu cubes, drain the tofu and cut it into finger-thick slices. Place the slices between sheets of kitchen paper and squeeze out the remaining liquid, then cut them into uniform cubes. Transfer the cubes to a bowl, add the cornflour and mix until all the cubes are well coated. Heat 1 tablespoon of oil in a non-stick frying pan and fry the tofu cubes on all sides until crispy and golden brown.

For the bowl, wash, trim and cut the cucumber, carrot and spring onion into thin sticks of uniform length. Wash and halve the tomato, then cut the halves into wedges. Clean and shred the red cabbage, then drizzle with the vinegar and knead briefly.

Optionally, you can make avocado roses. To do this, halve the avocado, remove the stone and carefully scoop the flesh out of the skin in one piece. One at a time, place a half-avocado on a lightly moistened work surface cut-side down and cut crossways into thin slices (the thinner the slices, the more delicate the rose). Using your hands, separate the slices and arrange them overlapping into a long line. Then carefully roll up the slices to form a rose.

When ready to serve, divide the rice, fried tofu cubes, vegetables, edamame, wakame salad and pickled ginger between two bowls. Then arrange an avocado rose in the middle of each bowl. Add toppings of your choice to the bowls, drizzle with soy sauce and serve.

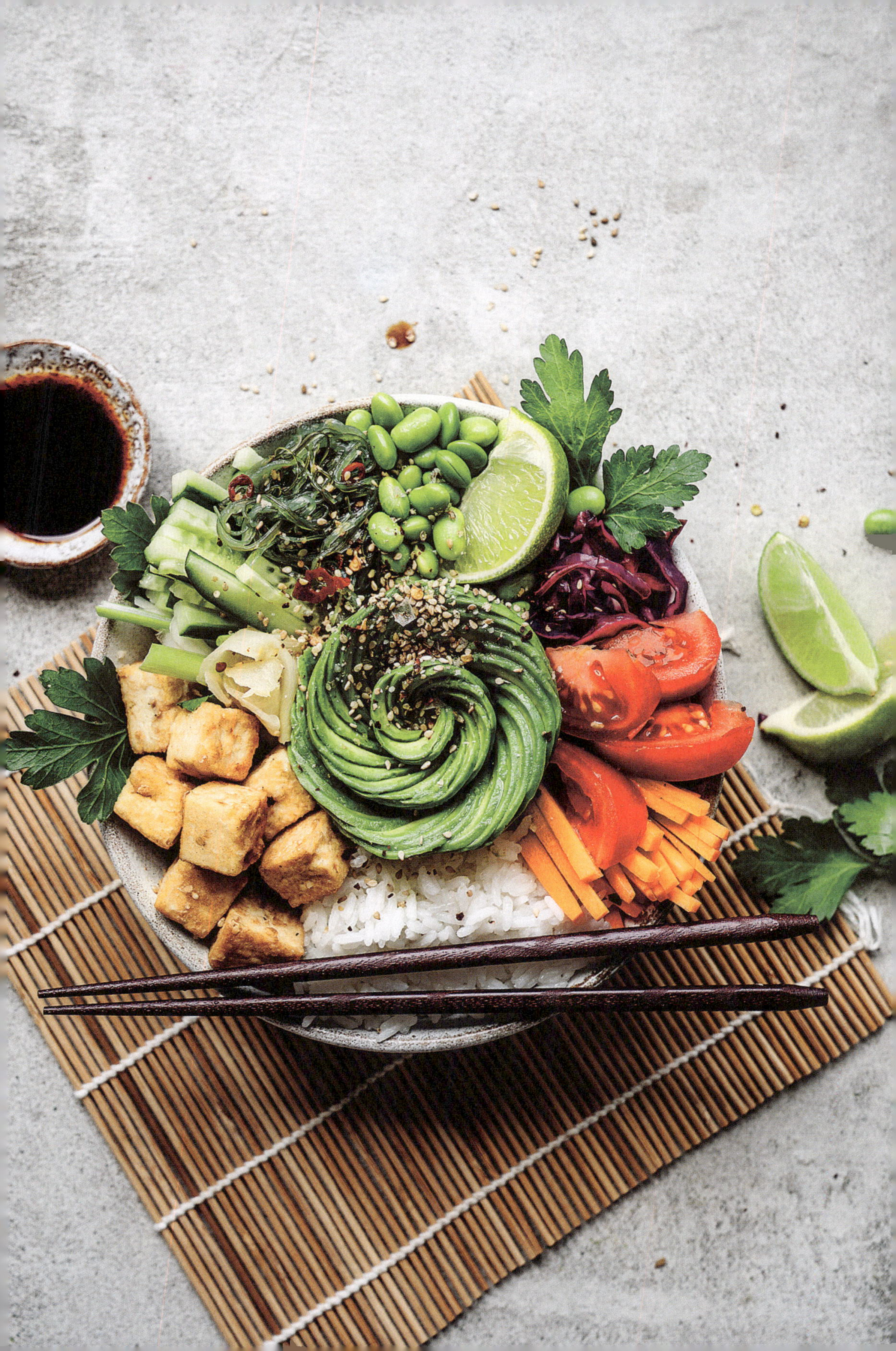

FALAFEL BOWL

FOR 2 BOWLS

FOR THE FALAFELS *(makes 12)*
200 g dried chickpeas, soaked for 12 hours
1 small onion
2 cloves garlic
½ bunch flat-leaf parsley
½ bunch coriander (optional)
1 tsp ground cumin
½ tsp ground coriander
½ tsp cayenne pepper
1 tsp sea salt
1–2 tbsp chickpea flour (as needed)
Sesame seeds
Olive oil

FOR THE TABBOULEH
75 g bulgur wheat
2 vine tomatoes
½ small onion
1 bunch flat-leaf parsley
2 tbsp freshly squeezed lemon juice
1 tbsp olive oil
Sea salt, freshly ground pepper

FOR THE RED CABBAGE AND SESAME SLAW
120 g red cabbage, shredded
1 tbsp rice vinegar
2 tsp sesame seeds
½ tsp agave syrup
Sea salt

FOR THE BOWL
2 handfuls baby spinach, cleaned
2 tbsp hummus (see page 119)
1 avocado
1 tbsp sesame seeds

EXTRAS
Toppings of your choice (e.g. chickpeas, pomegranate seeds, lime, coriander)
Olive oil

To make the falafel, place the chickpeas in a sieve, rinse thoroughly under running water and allow to drain. Peel the onion and garlic and coarsely chop them together with the parsley and coriander. Transfer the chickpeas to a blender, add all the other ingredients (except the chickpea flour) and blend to a slightly grainy paste. Transfer to a bowl and place in the fridge for at least 2 hours (or longer if desired) for the flavour to develop.

To make the tabbouleh, put the bulgur wheat into a bowl, add plenty of boiling water, cover and leave to soak for 30 minutes. In the meantime, wash and halve the tomatoes, then cut off the stem end, de-seed and cut into small dice. Peel the onion and finely chop together with the parsley. Mix everything together in a large salad bowl. Transfer the bulgur wheat to a sieve, refresh under cold running water and allow to drain. Add to the tomato mixture. Drizzle with the lemon juice and oil and mix well. Season with salt and pepper and set aside.

To make the red cabbage and sesame slaw, put all the ingredients into a bowl and knead them with your hands for 30 seconds.

Preheat the oven to 200°C. Take the falafel mixture out of the fridge and shape it into twelve balls. The falafels should hold together just enough to keep them moist when cooked. Add a little chickpea flour if necessary. Roll the falafels in the sesame seeds, arrange them on a baking tray lined with baking paper and bake for about 25 minutes. Turn them over after 15 minutes and brush them all over with a little olive oil.

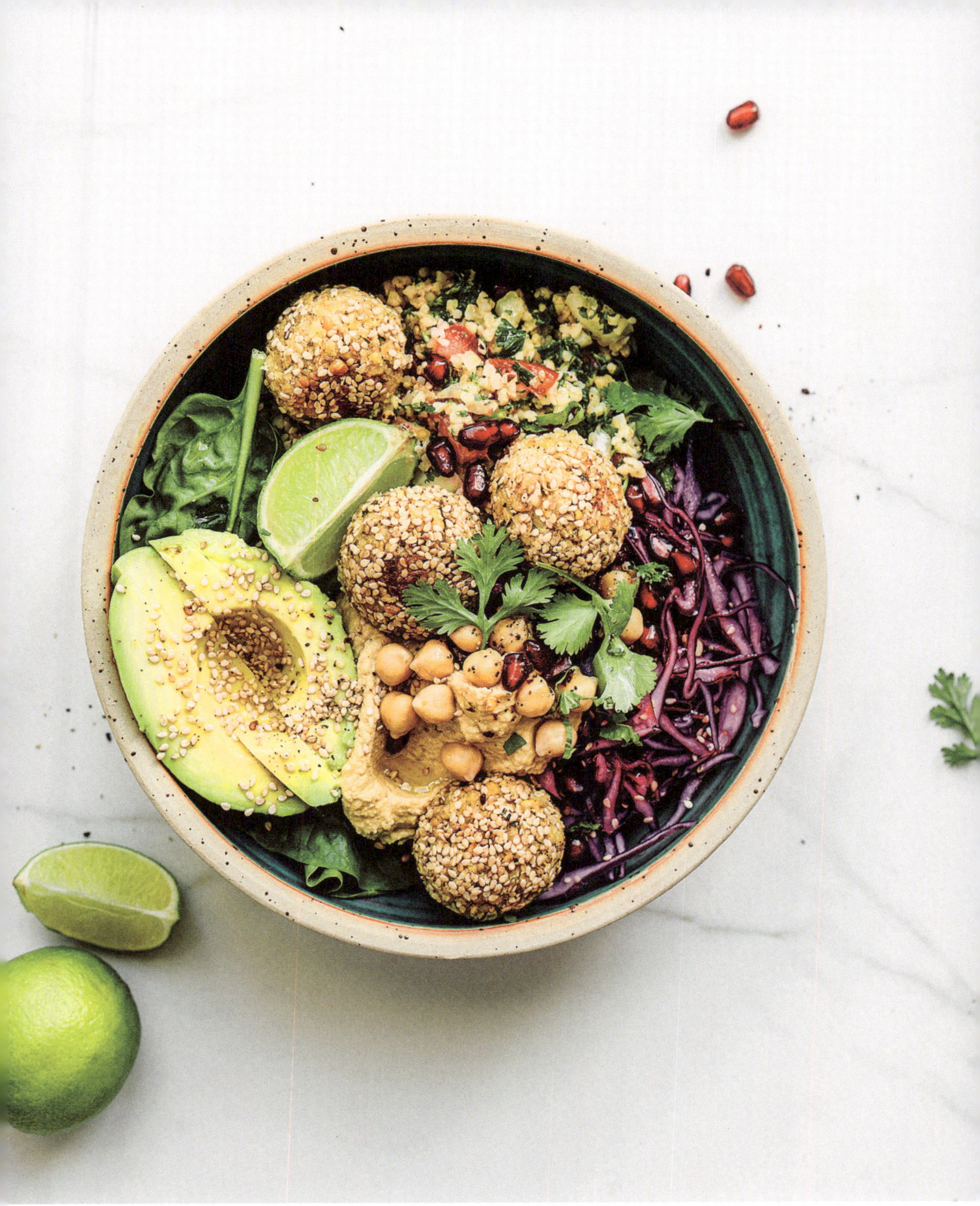

When ready to serve, divide the tabouleh, red cabbage and sesame slaw, baby spinach, hummus and four to six falafels between two bowls. Halve the avocado, remove the stone and score the flesh lengthways a few times. Using a spoon, scoop out the flesh and divide it between the bowls. Sprinkle with the sesame seeds, add the toppings of your choice, drizzle with olive oil and serve.

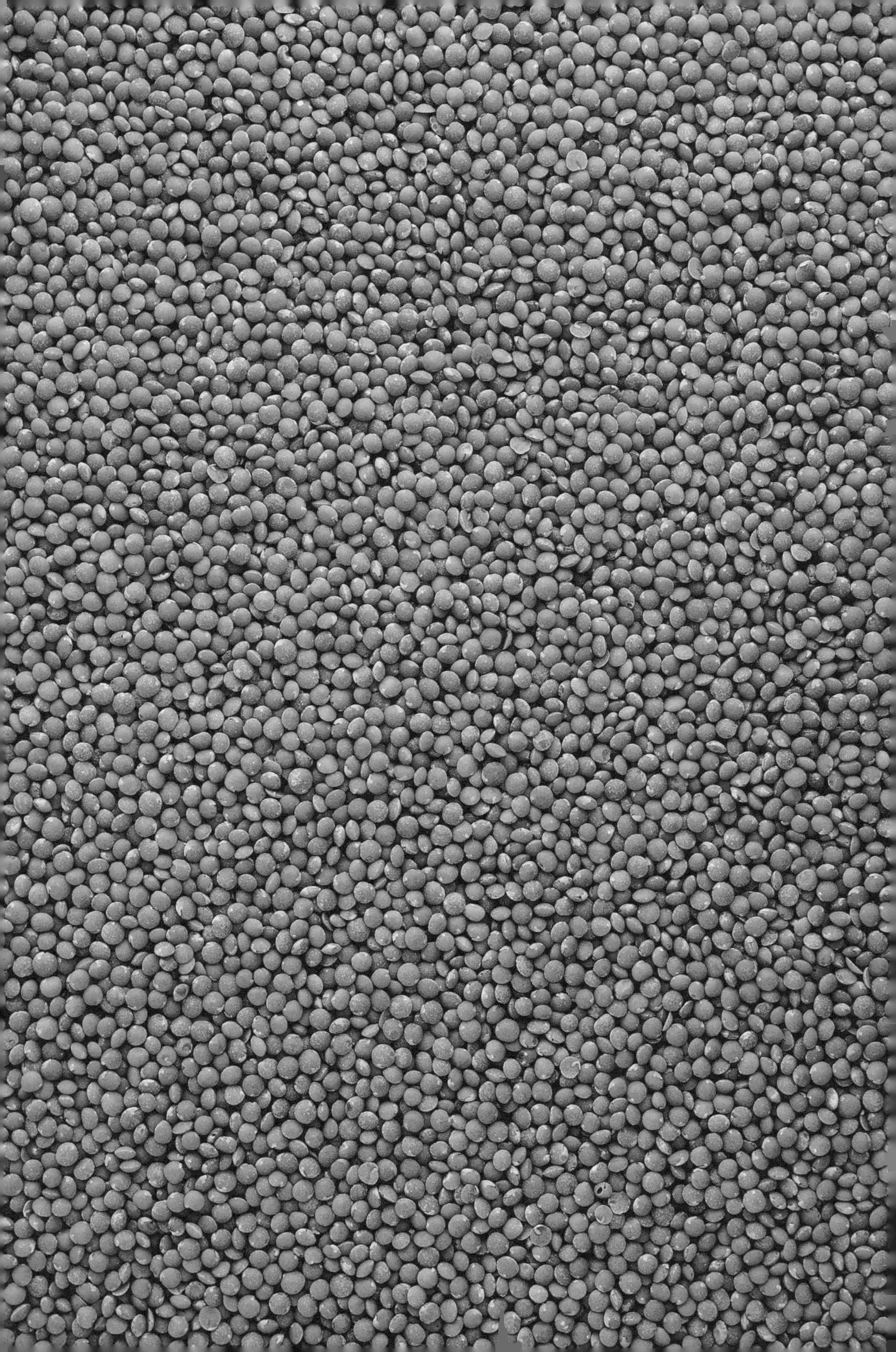

MAINS

With dishes to suit every occasion and preference – whether Italian, Asian, Indian, or Mexican – the colours and variety of plant-based cuisine are easy to see. Make boring meals a thing of the past.

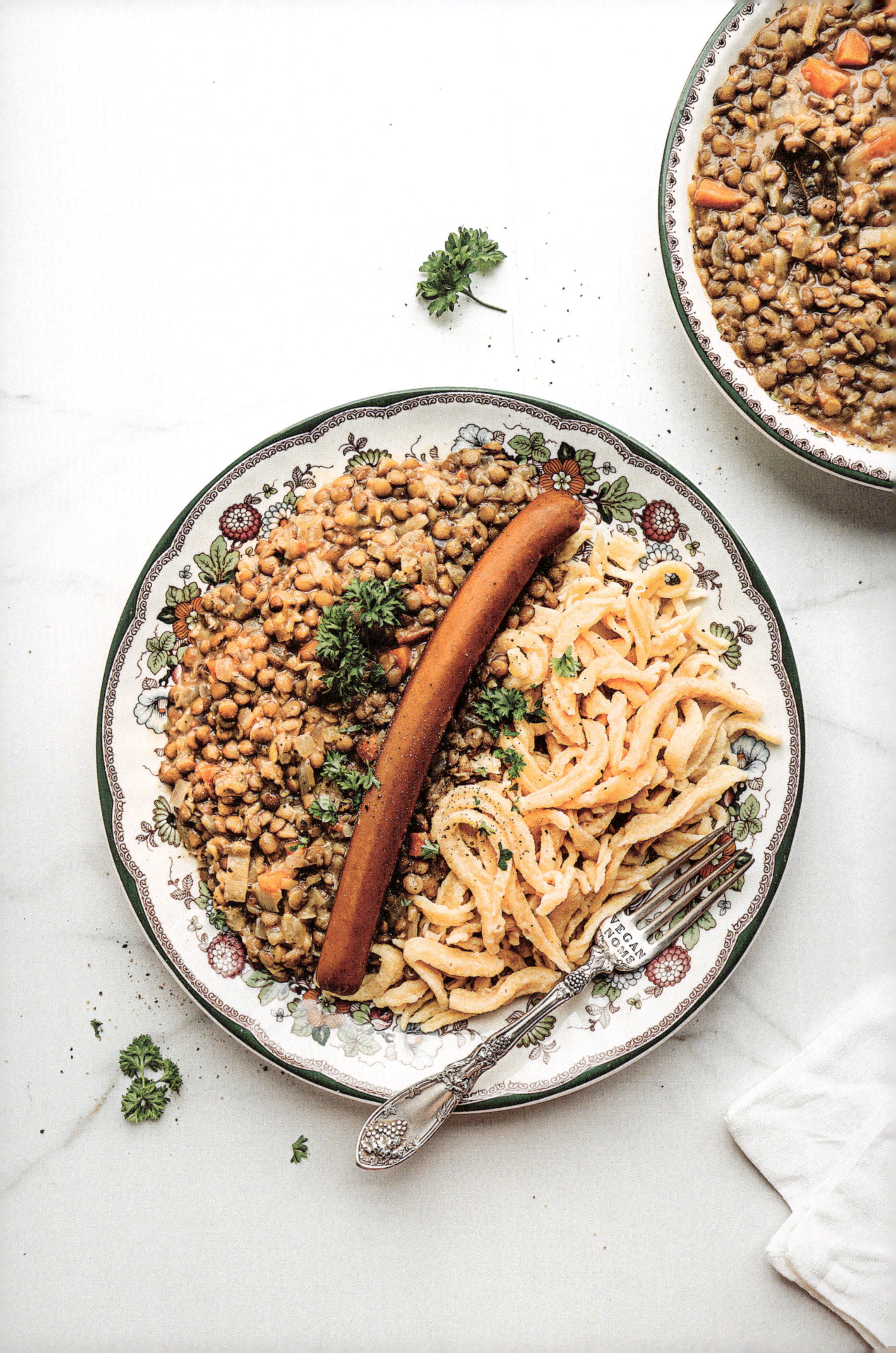
VEGAN
NOMS

LENTILS WITH SPELT SPAETZLE AND TOFU FRANKFURTERS

SERVES 2

FOR THE SPELT SPAETZLE

200 g wholemeal spelt flour
4 tbsp spelt semolina
1 tsp sea salt
1 pinch of ground turmeric
250 ml sparkling mineral water
1 tsp rapeseed oil, plus more for greasing

FOR THE LENTILS

150 g brown lentils, soaked overnight
1 carrot
½ leek
1 onion
1 bay leaf
1–2 tbsp plant-based margarine
1 tbsp wholemeal spelt flour
2 tbsp balsamic vinegar
Sea salt, freshly ground pepper

EXTRAS

2–4 tofu Frankfurters (quantity as desired)
Curly parsley, picked

To make the spelt spaetzle noodles, mix the dry ingredients together in a mixing bowl. Add the mineral water and oil and mix everything by hand or in a stand mixer until the mixture forms a viscous dough that falls off a spoon very slowly. Allow the dough to rest for about 20 minutes.

In the meantime, prepare and cook the lentils. Place the soaked lentils in a sieve, rinse thoroughly under running water and allow to drain. Clean and trim the carrot and leek, peel the onion, then cut everything separately into small dice. Put the lentils into a pan with the diced carrots, bay leaf and 500 ml of water and bring to the boil, then reduce the heat to low, cover and allow to simmer for 15 minutes. Drain the cooked lentils in a sieve and collect the cooking water. Discard the bay leaf.

Melt the margarine in a large pan and sauté the onion and leek. Stir in the flour and toast lightly. Deglaze the pan with a little lentil cooking water, stir and briefly bring to the boil. Then add the lentil and carrot mixture and the remaining cooking water to the pan and season with vinegar, salt and pepper. Adjust the amount of liquid as needed.

Bring salted water to the boil in a large pan, then reduce the heat (the water should be at a simmer not a rolling boil). Moisten a spaetzle board or a small chopping board with water, place some of dough on it and spread it out thinly with a dough scraper. Hold the board at an angle over the pan and scrape portions of the dough into long and thin noodles and allow them to fall into the water. Dip the dough scraper into the water from time to time to keep the dough from sticking. Allow the noodles to float to the surface and then remove them with a slotted spoon. Drain the spaetzle well and keep warm in a lightly greased dish until ready to serve.

Heat the tofu frankfurters in hot water. Arrange the frankfurters with portions of spaetzle and lentils on plates, garnish with parsley and serve.

• NOTE •

The spaetzle can easily be made in advance: simply make the dough according to the basic recipe (preferably double the amount). After cooking, transfer the noodles to a sieve, rinse briefly under cold water and allow to drain. Place in a bowl, drizzle with a little oil and store airtight in the fridge, or freeze in portions.

QUICK ONE-POT PASTA

SERVES 2

FOR THE PASTA

1 onion
2 cloves garlic
½ courgette
1 red pepper
1 carrot
100 g cherry vine tomatoes
200 g conchiglie (or orreccihette, farfalle or another type of short pasta)
400 g tinned chopped tomatoes
300 ml vegetable stock
200 ml coconut milk (at least 60% coconut extract)
150 g frozen peas
Sea salt, freshly ground pepper

EXTRAS

Cashew parmesan (see recipe on page 116)
Curly parsley, picked

Peel and finely chop the onion and garlic. Wash and trim the vegetables. Cut the courgettes and peppers into finger-thick chunks, quarter the carrot lengthways and dice, and halve the tomatoes.

Put the onion, garlic and vegetables into a pan with the pasta, tinned tomatoes, vegetable stock and coconut milk and bring to the boil. Reduce the heat and allow to simmer gently, uncovered, for 10 minutes. Gently mix in the peas and cook for a further 3–5 minutes until the pasta is cooked and the sauce thickens to a creamy consistency. Stir from time to time to ensure even cooking.

Season the pasta with salt and pepper, top with cashew parmesan, garnish with parsley and serve.

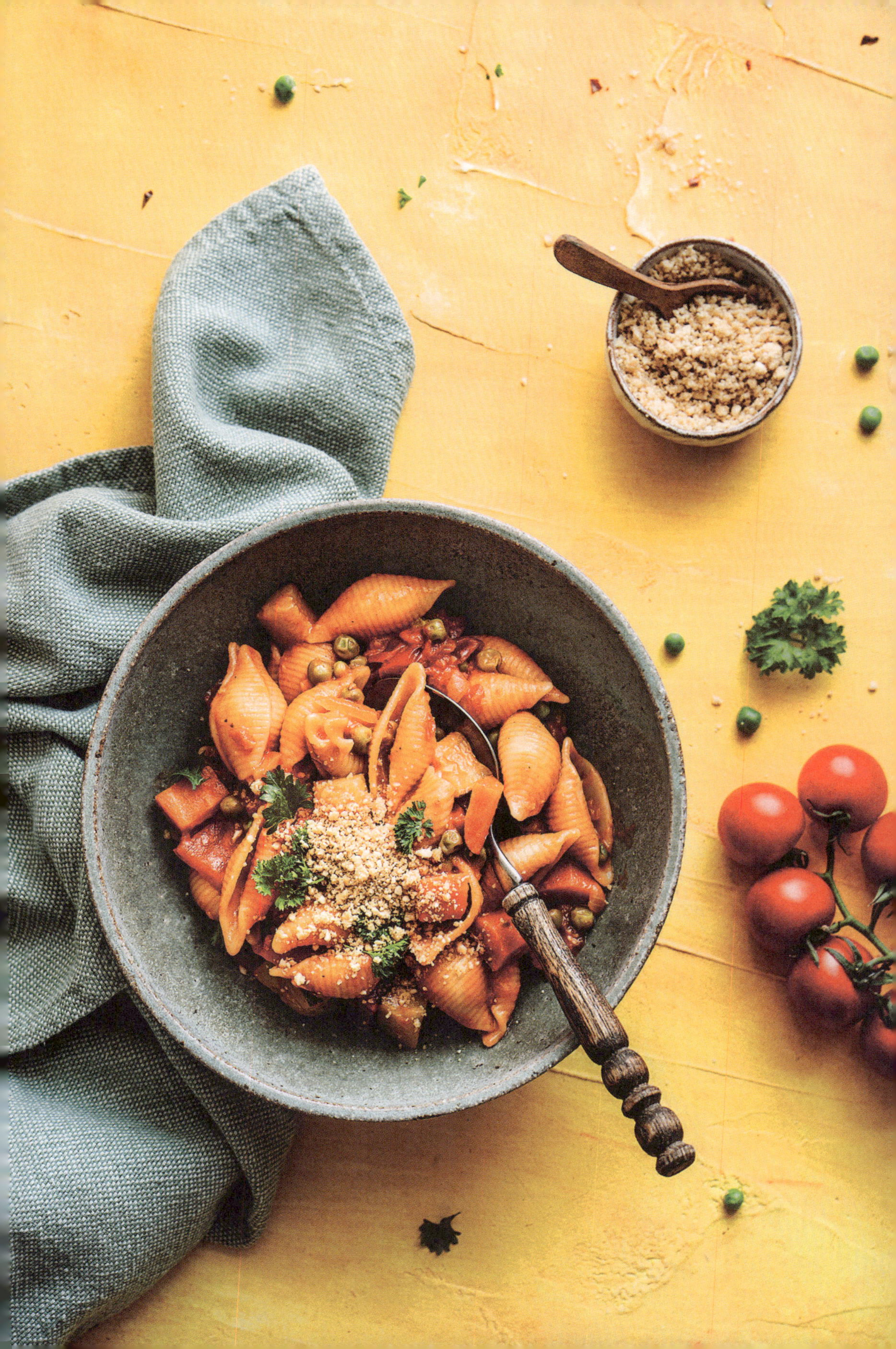

RICOTTA & SPINACH RAVIOLI WITH SAGE BUTTER

SERVES 4

FOR THE DOUGH
150 g wholemeal spelt flour, plus more for dusting
150 g durum wheat semolina
½ tsp sea salt
1 pinch of ground turmeric

FOR THE FILLING
200 g firm tofu
1 clove garlic
2 tbsp yeast flakes
1 tbsp almond butter
2 tsp apple cider vinegar
1 tsp freshly squeezed lemon juice
½ tsp sea salt
200 g frozen spinach, thawed
Freshly ground pepper, freshly grated nutmeg

FOR THE SAGE BUTTER
1–2 clove(s) garlic
10 sage leaves
50 g plant-based margarine

To make the dough, mix all the ingredients in a bowl, add 150 ml cold water and knead the mixture with your hands for 10 minutes, until the dough is firm and smooth. Wrap the dough in cling film and allow to rest in the fridge for 1 hour.

For the filling, drain the tofu and mash in a bowl with a fork. Peel and finely chop the garlic and add it to the tofu. Add the yeast flakes, almond butter, vinegar, lemon juice and sea salt to the tofu and mix well until combined. Squeeze any liquid out of the thawed spinach and chop finely. Mix the spinach into the tofu mixture and season with pepper and nutmeg.

To make the ravioli, lightly dust the work surface with flour and roll out the pasta dough very thinly using a rolling pin. Use a biscuit cutter or round object (e.g. a glass) to cut out 8-cm-diameter discs. Place a tablespoon of the filling in the centre of half the dough discs and brush all around with water to moisten the dough. Cover with another dough disc and seal by carefully pressing the edges down using your thumb or a fork.

Bring salted water to a simmer (not a rolling boil) in a large pan and cook the ravioli in batches for 4–6 minutes, until they float to the surface. Then remove with a slotted spoon and drain.

To make the sage butter, peel and thinly slice the garlic. Wash the sage and carefully pat dry. Melt the margarine in a frying pan and lightly sauté the garlic and sage.

When ready to serve, toss the drained ravioli in the hot sage butter and serve immediately.

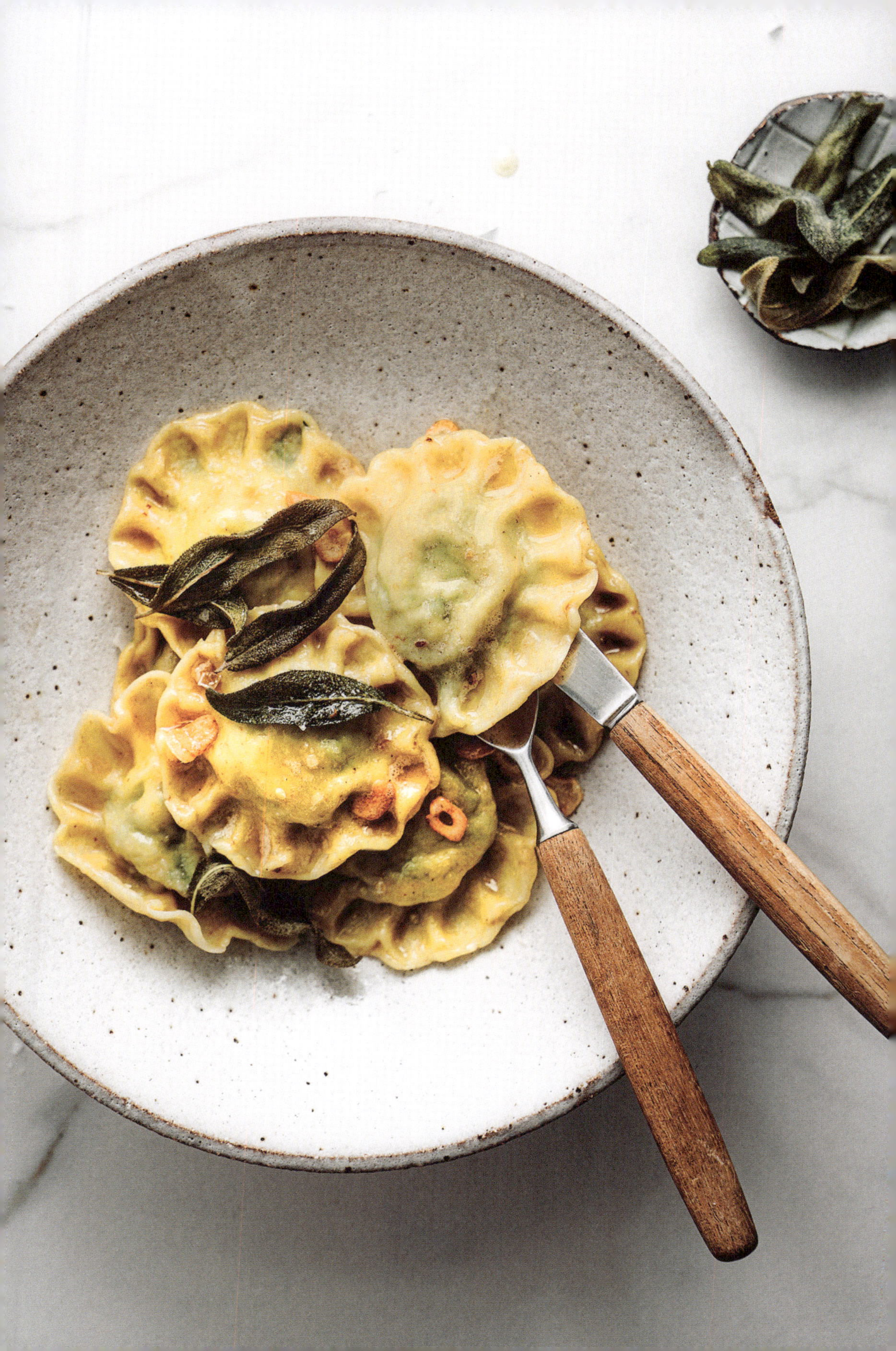

TERIYAKI TEMPEH AND NOODLE STIR-FRY

SERVES 4

FOR THE TEMPEH

200 g tempeh
3 cloves garlic, crushed
2 tbsp soy sauce
1 tbsp balsamic vinegar
1 tbsp agave syrup

FOR THE STIR-FRY

200 g mie noodles
½ head broccoli
2 carrots
1 small courgette
2 spring onions
1 red pepper
1 green pepper
100 g mangetout
2 cloves garlic
1 thumb-sized piece of ginger (30 g when peeled)
100 g bamboo shoots
100 g mung bean sprouts
2 tbsp peanut oil (or rapeseed oil)

FOR THE TERIYAKI SAUCE

50 ml soy sauce
2 tbsp agave syrup
1 tbsp rice vinegar
2 tbsp sesame seeds
1 tbsp cornflour

Cut the tempeh into bite-sized chunks. Mix the remaining ingredients together in a bowl, then add the tempeh, coat well and marinate in the fridge for 1 hour (or longer if desired).

Cook the noodles according to the packet instructions. Transfer the noodles to a sieve, refresh in cold water and allow to drain. Set aside.

Wash and trim the vegetables. Then divide the broccoli into florets, slice the carrots and courgettes slightly on a diagonal, halve the spring onions and quarter them lengthways, and cut the peppers into strips. Leave the mangetout whole. Peel and finely chop the garlic and ginger. Place the bean sprouts in a sieve, rinse thoroughly under running water and allow to drain.

Heat 1 tablespoon of oil in a wok or large non-stick frying pan. Take the tempeh out of the marinade and stir-fry in the hot oil until crispy, then remove and set aside. Add the remaining tablespoon of oil to the wok and stir-fry the carrots over a high heat for 2 minutes. Add the broccoli, peppers, courgette, ginger and garlic and stir-fry for 3–5 minutes. Reduce the heat, then add the spring onions, mangetout, bamboo shoots and bean sprouts and briefly sauté together. The vegetables should be cooked through but still crisp and firm to the bite.

To make the teriyaki sauce, put the soy sauce, agave syrup, rice vinegar, sesame seeds and 100 ml of water into a small pan and bring to the boil. Make a slurry by mixing the cornflour with 2 tablespoons of cold water and stir it into the mixture in the pan. Bring the sauce back to the boil while stirring until thickened.

When ready to serve, pour the teriyaki sauce over the stir-fried vegetables, fold in the noodles and tempeh and serve hot.

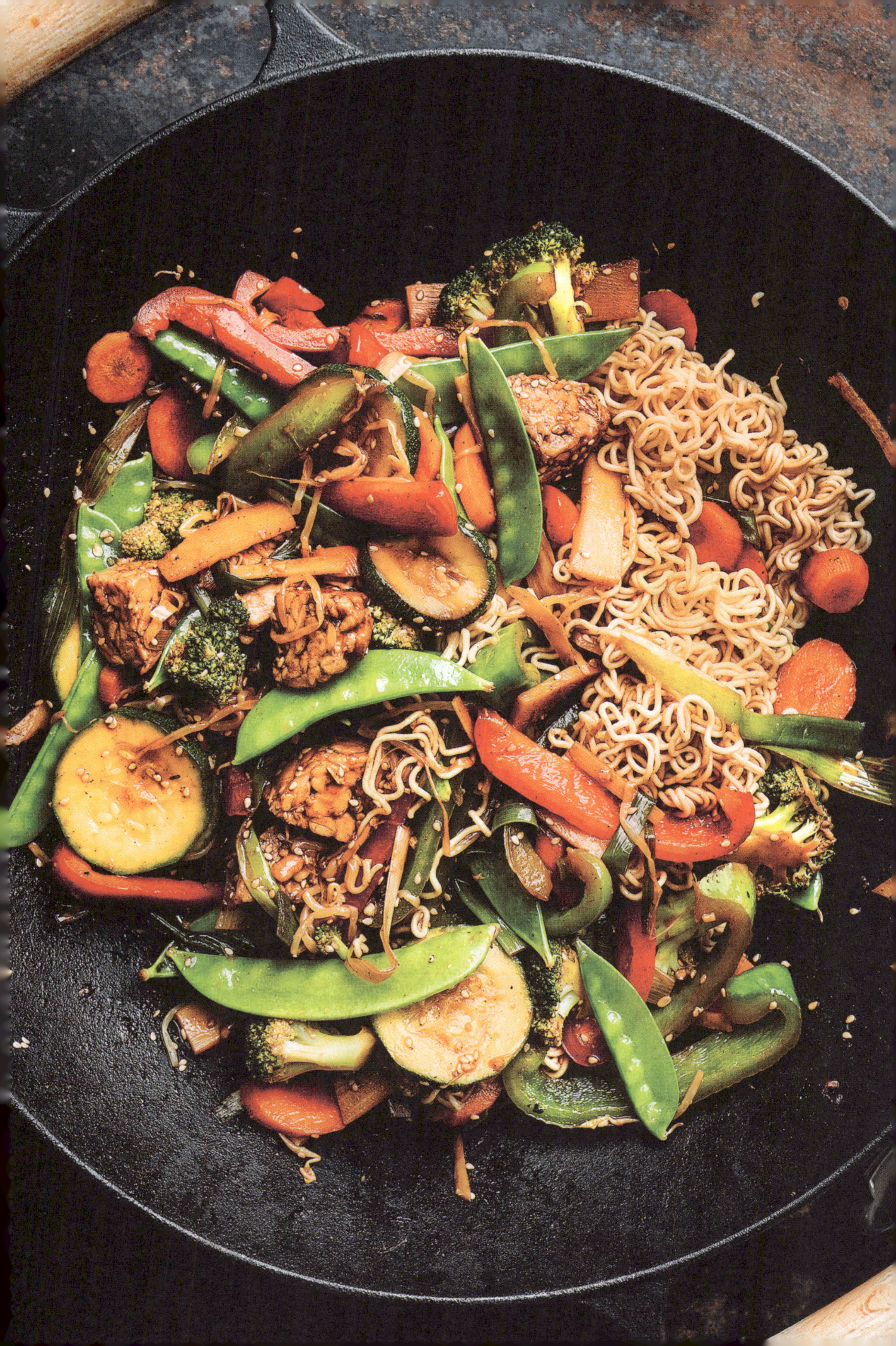

SATAY TOFU SKEWERS WITH LIME RICE

SERVES 2

FOR THE RED CURRY PASTE *(makes 250 ml)*
1 onion
6 cloves garlic
1 thumb-sized piece of ginger (30 g when peeled)
1 stalk lemongrass
4 Thai chilli peppers (available from Oriental supermarkets)
2 tbsp coconut oil, melted
2 tbsp sweet paprika
1 tbsp chopped coriander leaves (optional)
1 tbsp sugar
1 tsp untreated lime zest
1 tsp ground cumin
1 tsp ground coriander
1 tsp sea salt

FOR THE TOFU SKEWERS *(4 pieces)*
200 g firm tofu
1 tbsp soy sauce
1 tbsp agave syrup
2 tsp red curry paste
4 pepper wedges (all one colour or different colours)
1 tbsp rapeseed oil

FOR THE LIME RICE
200 g jasmine rice
2 tbsp freshly squeezed lime juice
1 tsp untreated lime zest
1–2 tbsp chopped coriander leaves
Sea salt

FOR THE SATAY SAUCE
80 g roasted and salted peanuts
200 ml coconut milk (at least 60% coconut extract)
1–2 tbsp red curry paste
2 tsp freshly squeezed lemon juice
1 tsp agave syrup

EXTRAS
Toppings of your choice (e.g. coriander, lime, chopped peanuts)

To make the red curry paste, peel the onion and garlic, peel the ginger and clean and trim the lemongrass. Coarsely chop everything. Wash the chillies, remove the stems and coarsely chop. Put all the ingredients into a mixing beaker and blend to a paste using a stick blender. Transfer the curry paste to a screw-top jar and set aside.

To make the tofu skewers, drain the tofu and cut it into cubes. Mix the soy sauce, agave syrup and curry paste together in a bowl, then add the tofu, coat well and marinate in the fridge for 1 hour (or longer if desired). Cut the pepper wedges into pieces (no larger than the tofu cubes) and set aside.

To make the lime rice, cook the jasmine rice according to the packet instructions. Fold in the remaining ingredients and season to taste.

To make the satay sauce, finely grind the peanuts in a blender. Heat 50 ml of coconut milk in a small pan and reduce until fragrant. Gently stir in the curry paste and cook for 1–2 minutes. Add the ground peanuts and remaining 150 ml of coconut milk and cook, stirring constantly, until the sauce has thickened enough to coat the back of a spoon. Remove from the heat and adjust the flavour with lemon juice and agave syrup, seasoning if necessary.

Next, prepare the tofu skewers. Remove the tofu from the marinade and thread the cubes onto bamboo skewers, alternating with the pieces of pepper. Heat the oil in a non-stick frying pan, add the skewers and cook until golden brown all over.

When ready to serve, divide the lime rice and the tofu skewers between two bowls. Serve with the satay sauce and toppings of your choice.

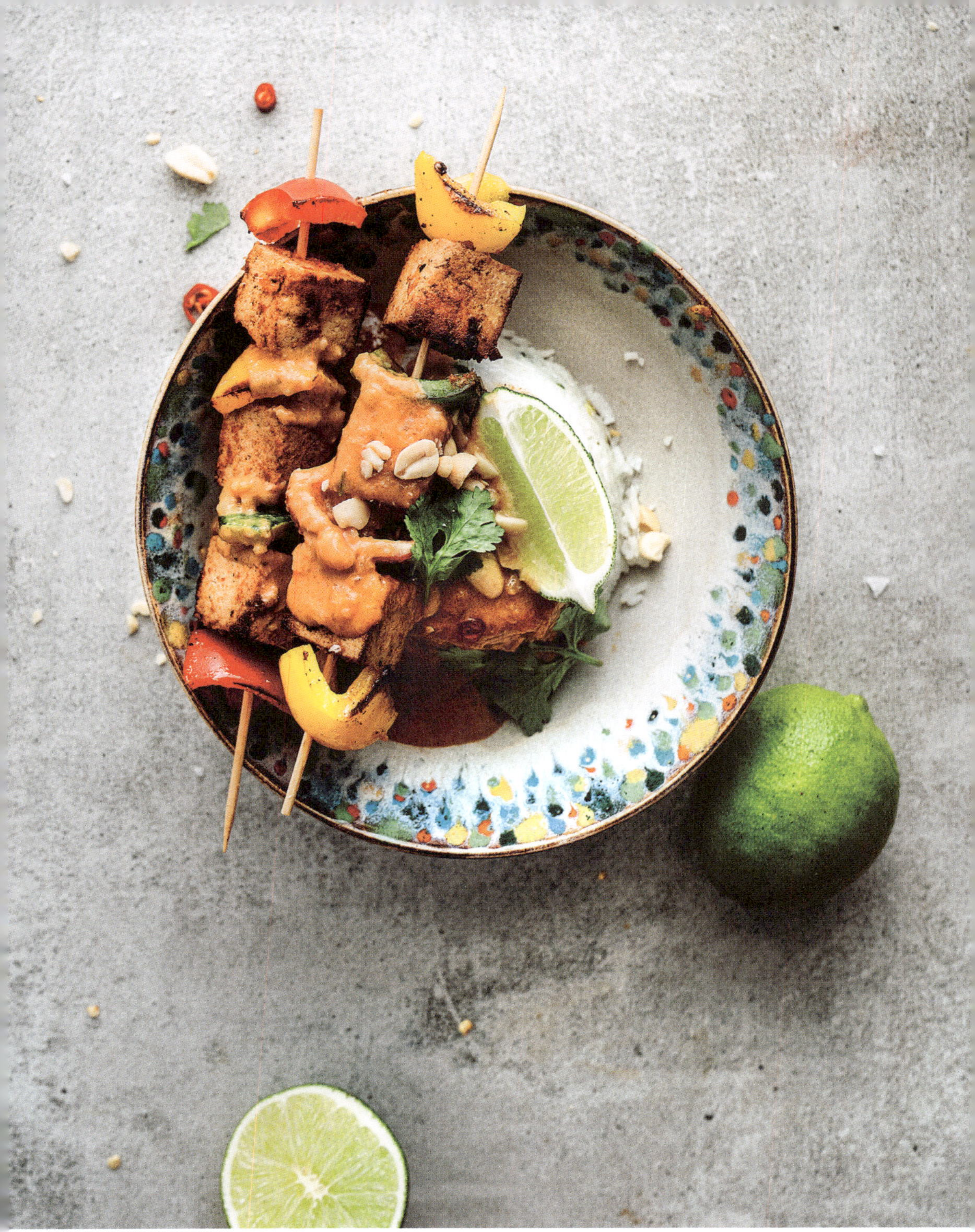

• NOTE •

If stored in an airtight container in the fridge, the curry paste will keep for several weeks. You can also divide it into portions (e.g. in an ice tray) and freeze it. This will allow you to always have some to hand and make a big difference to the way you cook.

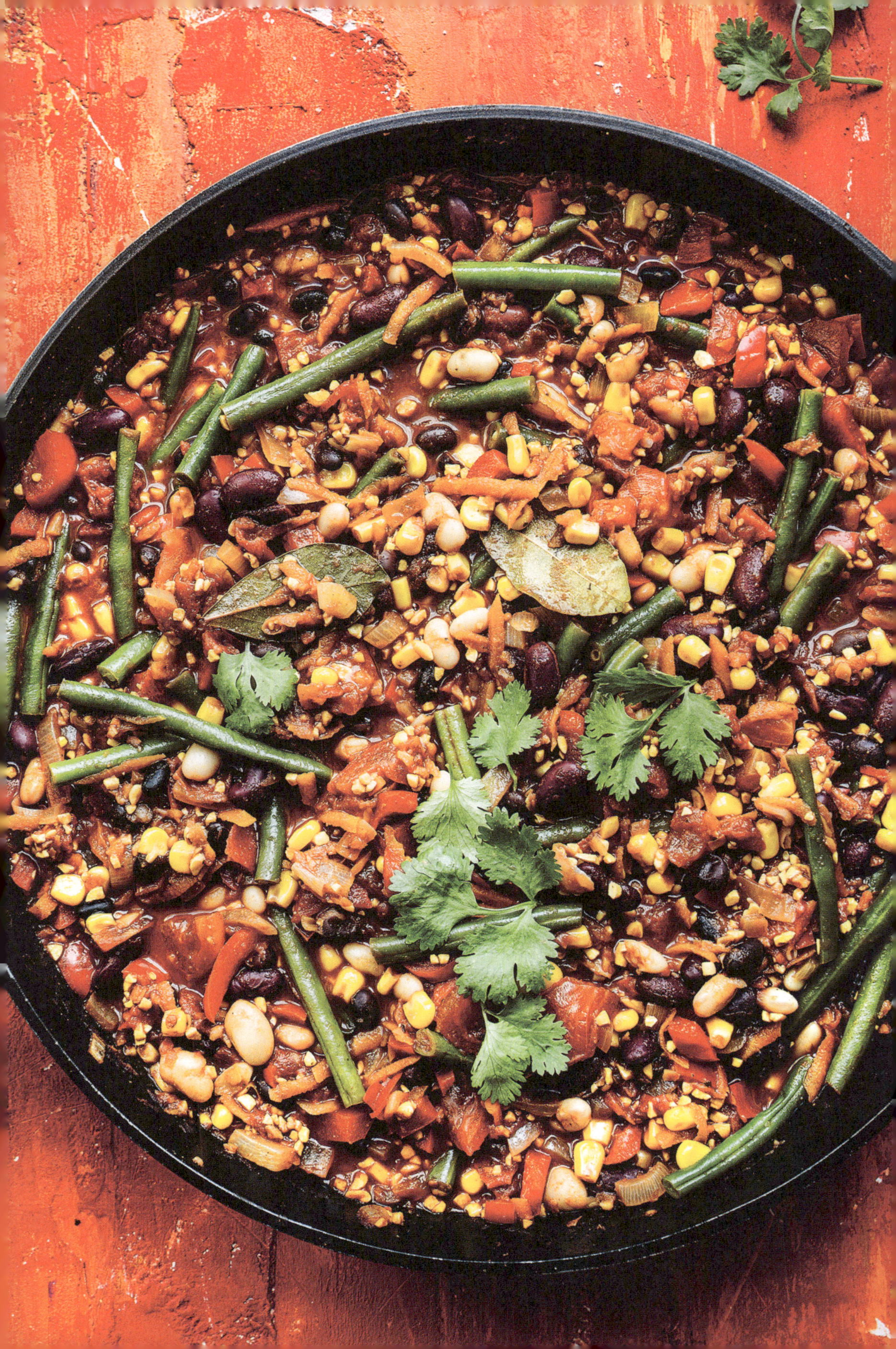

FIERY FOUR-BEAN CHILLI

SERVES 4

FOR THE CHILLI
100 g lupin groats
2 medium onions
3 cloves garlic
3 vine tomatoes
1 red pepper
1 medium carrot
1 tbsp rapeseed oil
1 tbsp chilli powder
2 tsp sweet paprika
1 tsp ground cumin
1 tbsp cocoa powder
4 tbsp tomato purée
1 tbsp agave syrup
400 g tinned chopped tomatoes
400 ml vegetable stock
2 bay leaves
150 g dwarf French beans
150 g cooked kidney beans
150 g cooked white beans
150 g cooked black beans
1 tin sweetcorn (140 g drained weight)
2 tbsp freshly squeezed lemon juice
Sea salt

EXTRAS
Accompaniment of your choice (e.g. basmati rice, flatbread)
Toppings of your choice (e.g. ripe avocado, coriander)

Put the lupin groats into a small pan, cover with water and simmer for 5 minutes. Then turn off the heat, cover and allow the pan to stand on the still-warm hob for 15 minutes. Transfer the lupin groats to a sieve, rinse thoroughly and allow to drain.

Peel and finely chop the onions and garlic. Wash the tomatoes and pepper, then trim and finely dice. Peel and grate the carrot.

Heat the oil in a large frying pan and sauté the lupin groats with the onions over a high heat. Add the garlic, spices and cocoa powder and allow the spices to toast for 30 seconds while stirring constantly. Stir in the tomato purée and agave syrup and cook briefly to caramelise. Then add the tomatoes, peppers and grated carrots to the pan, deglaze with the tinned tomatoes and vegetable stock and stir well. Add the bay leaves, cover the pan and allow the chilli to cook over a medium heat for 15 minutes, stirring from time to time. If the chilli becomes too thick, add more liquid.

In the meantime, wash, trim and halve the green beans. Place all the cooked beans and sweetcorn in a sieve, rinse thoroughly under running water and allow to drain. Add the green beans to the chilli and continue to cook for a further 15 minutes. After about 10 minutes, stir the bean mixture and the sweetcorn into the chilli.

Season the finished chilli with lemon juice and salt. Serve with accompaniments and toppings of your choice.

• NOTE •
For this recipe, you can also substitute the lupin groats with soya mince (TVP). In this case, simply put 100 g of soya mince in a bowl, cover with hot vegetable stock and allow to soak for 15 minutes. Then drain in a sieve and continue with the recipe instructions.

COLOURFUL LENTIL PANCAKES

SERVES 4

FOR THE PANCAKES
150 g red lentils
½ tsp sea salt

FOR THE TOPPING
250 g chestnut mushrooms
200 g cherry vine tomatoes
½ small red onion
4 lettuce leaves of your choice
200 g tempeh
2 tbsp soy sauce
1 tbsp agave syrup
1 tbsp sesame seeds
Rapeseed oil
1 avocado
Hummus (see page 119)

EXTRAS
Tahini sauce (see page 120, optional)

To make the pancakes, place the lentils in a sieve and rinse thoroughly under running water until the water runs clear. Transfer the lentils to a bowl, add 325 ml of water and soak them for at least 4 hours. Then transfer the soaked lentils to a blender, add the soaking water and salt and blend to a thick, mushy batter.

To make the topping, clean, trim and slice the mushrooms. Wash and halve the cherry tomatoes. Peel and slice the onion into thin rings. Wash the lettuce leaves and pat dry. Cut the tempeh into twelve slices. Mix the soy sauce, agave syrup and sesame seeds together in a small bowl.

Heat a dry non-stick frying pan and place a ladle of lentil batter in the centre. Using the bottom of the ladle and without pressing, spread the batter across the pan in a circular motion. Cook the batter for about 2 minutes over a medium heat, until the top becomes firm, then carefully turn the pancake over. Repeat the process with the remaining batter to make four pancakes. If the pancakes stick, brush the pan with a little oil. Transfer the pancakes to a plate, stacking each freshly made one on top of the others, and cover with a cloth to keep warm.

Heat 1 teaspoon of oil in the same pan and briefly sauté the mushrooms over a high heat, and remove them from the pan. Wipe the pan clean with kitchen paper, heat another tablespoon of oil and fry the tempeh slices on both sides until golden brown. Then remove the pan from the heat, allow it to stand for 1 minute and pour the soy sauce mixture over the tempeh. Return the pan to a low heat and allow the liquid to simmer while constantly turning the tempeh slices.

When ready to serve, halve the avocado, remove the stone, scoop out the flesh and cut it into thin wedges. Spread each lentil pancake with hummus and top with the vegetables, lettuce, avocado and sesame tempeh. Serve with tahini sauce if desired.

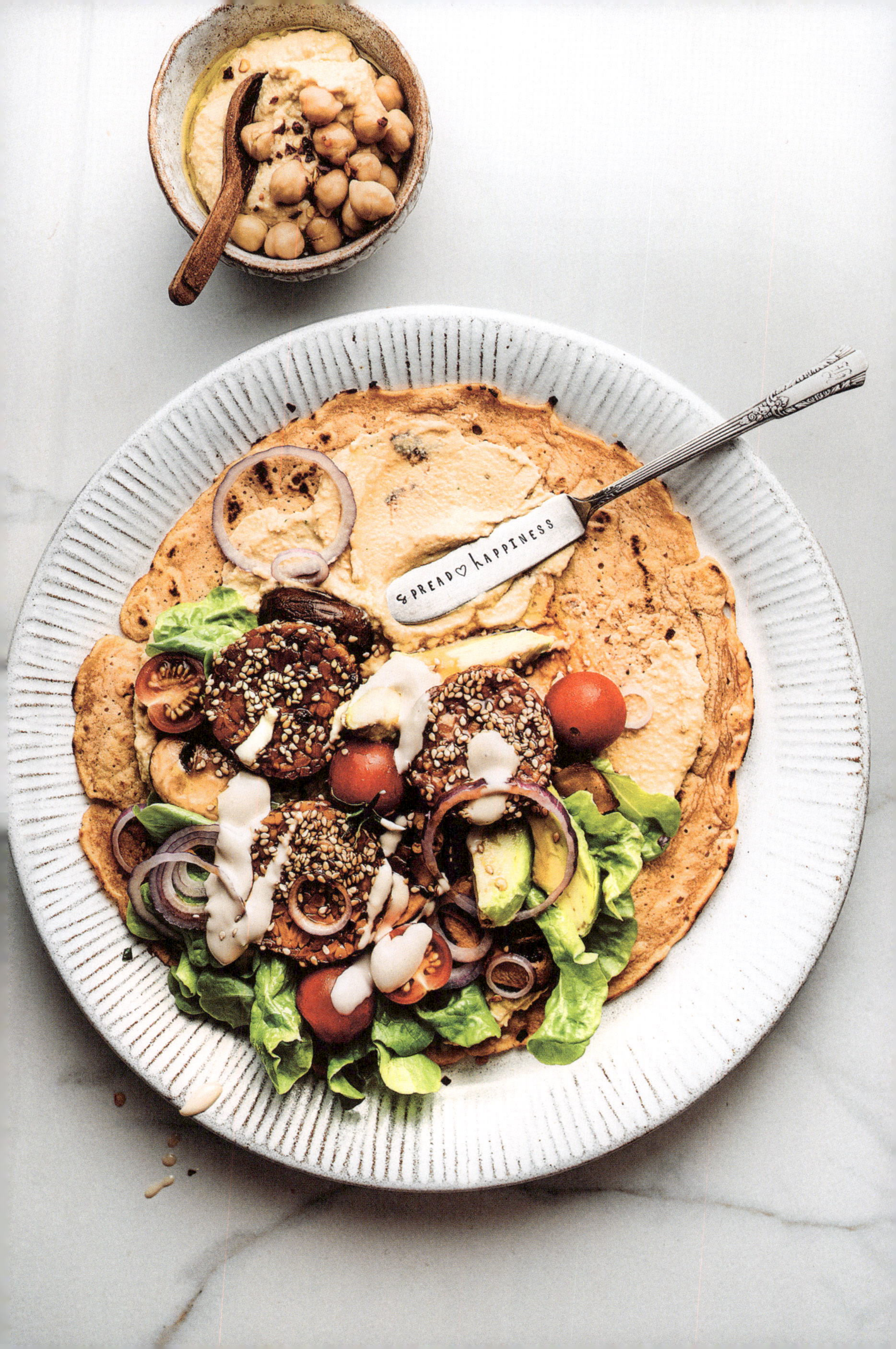
SPREAD♡HAPPINESS

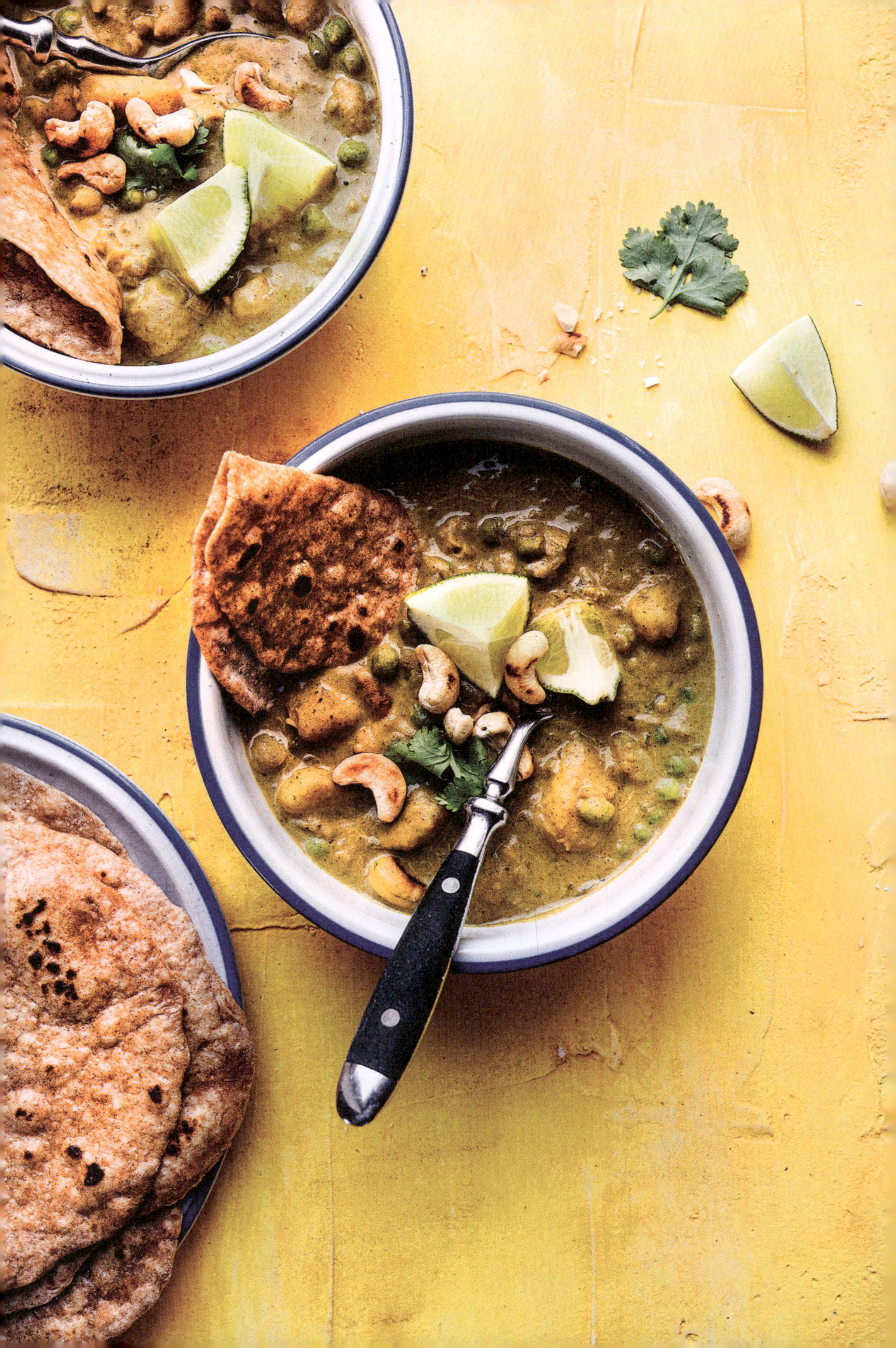

POTATO CURRY WITH WHOLEMEAL CHAPATIS

SERVES 4

FOR THE POTATO CURRY

800 g waxy potatoes (peeled before weighing)
2 medium onions
3 cloves garlic
1 tbsp coconut oil
2 tbsp freshly grated ginger
1½ tbsp garam masala
1 tsp ground coriander
1 tsp ground turmeric
1 tsp cayenne pepper
400 ml coconut milk (at least 60% coconut extract)
250 g frozen peas
2 tbsp freshly squeezed lime juice
Sea salt

FOR THE CHAPATIS *(makes 8)*

200 g wholemeal spelt flour, plus more for dusting
½ tsp sea salt
1 tbsp olive oil
Plant-based margarine

EXTRAS

2 handfuls cashew nuts
Toppings of your choice (e.g. coriander, lime)

To make the potato curry, peel the potatoes, quarter lengthways and cut them into pieces about 2.5-cm in size. Peel and finely chop the onions and garlic. Heat the coconut oil in a pan and sauté the onions until translucent. Add the garlic, ginger and spices and allow the spices to toast for 30 seconds while stirring constantly. Then add the potatoes to the pan with 800 ml of water. Bring to the boil, cover and cook over a medium heat for 10 minutes. Then remove the lid and cook for a further 10–15 minutes, until the potatoes are cooked through and the liquid is almost completely reduced. Stir regularly to keep the contents of the pan from burning. Add the coconut milk and frozen peas and continue to cook until the sauce thickens. Season with lime juice and salt.

To make the chapatis, mix the flour and salt in a bowl. Gradually mix in 125 ml of warm water and the oil and then knead the dough until smooth and supple. Cover the bowl with a clean cloth and allow the dough to rest for 10 minutes. Then divide the dough into eight portions. Lightly dust the work surface with flour and roll out each portion into a thin disc. Place a dry non-stick frying pan over a high heat and cook the chapatis for 20–30 seconds on each side. Transfer the finished chapatis to a plate, immediately brushing with a little margarine and covering with a clean cloth until ready to serve.

When ready to serve, add the cashews to the pan and lightly toast them over a low heat. Serve the potato curry with the wholemeal chapatis, toasted cashews and toppings of your choice.

AYURVEDIC KITCHARI

SERVES 4

FOR THE KITCHARI

200 g split mung beans (mung dal, available from organic food shops), soaked for at least 2 hours or overnight
100 g basmati rice
300 g carrots
1 thumb-sized piece of ginger (30 g when peeled)
1 tsp ground cumin
1 tsp ground coriander
1 tsp ground turmeric
½ tsp freshly ground pepper
⅓ tsp ground cinnamon
1 tbsp coconut oil
1 tsp black mustard seeds
1 tsp cumin seeds
2 tbsp freshly squeezed lime juice
Sea salt

EXTRAS

Toppings of your choice (e.g. chilli oil, coriander, lime)

Place the soaked mung beans and rice in a sieve, rinse thoroughly under running water and allow to drain. Peel and cut the carrots into about 1-cm dice. Peel and finely grate the ginger. Mix the ground spices in a small bowl.

Heat the coconut oil in a pan and toast the mustard seeds and cumin until fragrant (watch closely to keep from burning). Add the ginger and ground spices and allow the spices to toast for 30 seconds. Add the mung beans, rice and carrots to the pan, followed by 1 litre of water and mix well. Bring the kitchari to the boil, then reduce the heat to low and simmer gently for 15 minutes (without stirring). After the cooking time, remove the lid and continue to simmer for a further 5 minutes.

By this time, the water will have been almost completely absorbed and the rice and beans should be nice and soft. Adjust the amount of liquid depending on the desired consistency.

Season the kitchari with lime juice and salt and serve with toppings of your choice.

· NOTE ·

Not only is kitchari suitable for lunch or dinner, but it also makes a soothing and easily digestible breakfast in the morning. You can also make it with a lot of other great vegetables instead of carrots (e.g. sweet potatoes, celery, fennel, pumpkin or squash, spinach, Swiss chard). Let the season inspire your choice.

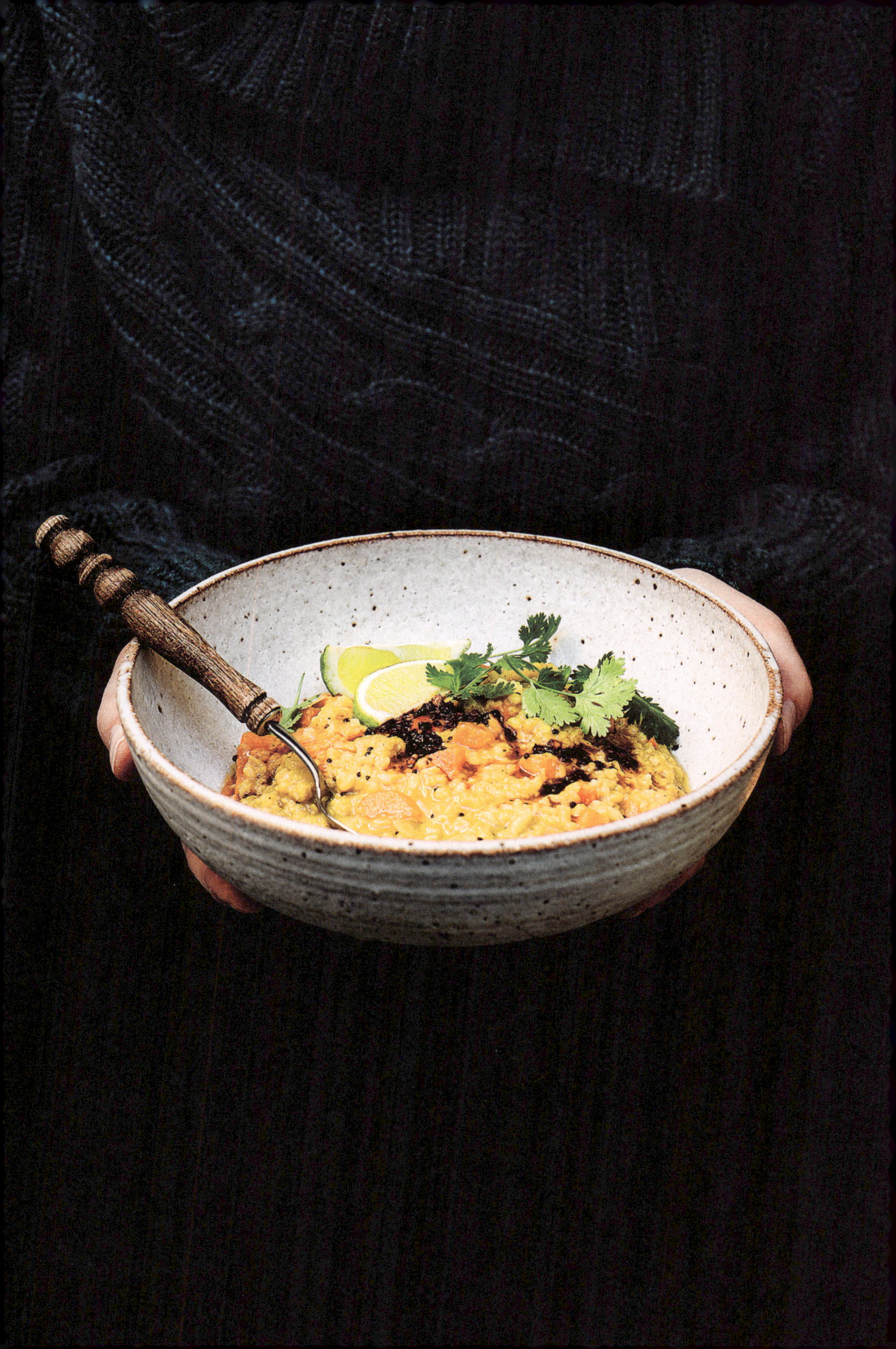

RED LENTIL DAL

SERVES 4

FOR THE DAL

1 medium onion
2 cloves garlic
1 thumb-sized piece of ginger (30 g when peeled)
1 tbsp coconut oil
2 tbsp desiccated coconut
1 tsp ground cumin
1 tsp ground turmeric
½ tsp ground coriander
200 g red lentils
400 g tinned chopped tomatoes
400 ml coconut milk (at least 60% coconut extract)
1–2 tbsp freshly squeezed lime juice
Sea salt, cayenne pepper

EXTRAS

Accompaniment of your choice (e.g. basmati rice, flatbread)
Toppings of your choice (e.g. coriander, lime)

Peel and finely chop the onion and garlic. Peel and finely grate the ginger.

Heat the coconut oil in a pan and sauté the onion until translucent. Then add the garlic, ginger, desiccated coconut and spices and allow the spices to toast for 30 seconds while stirring constantly. Add the lentils, tinned tomatoes and coconut milk. Cover the pan and gently simmer for 12–15 minutes, until the lentils are cooked.

Season with lime juice, salt and cayenne pepper. If the lentils absorb too much water, add a little more liquid. Serve the dal with accompaniments and toppings of your choice.

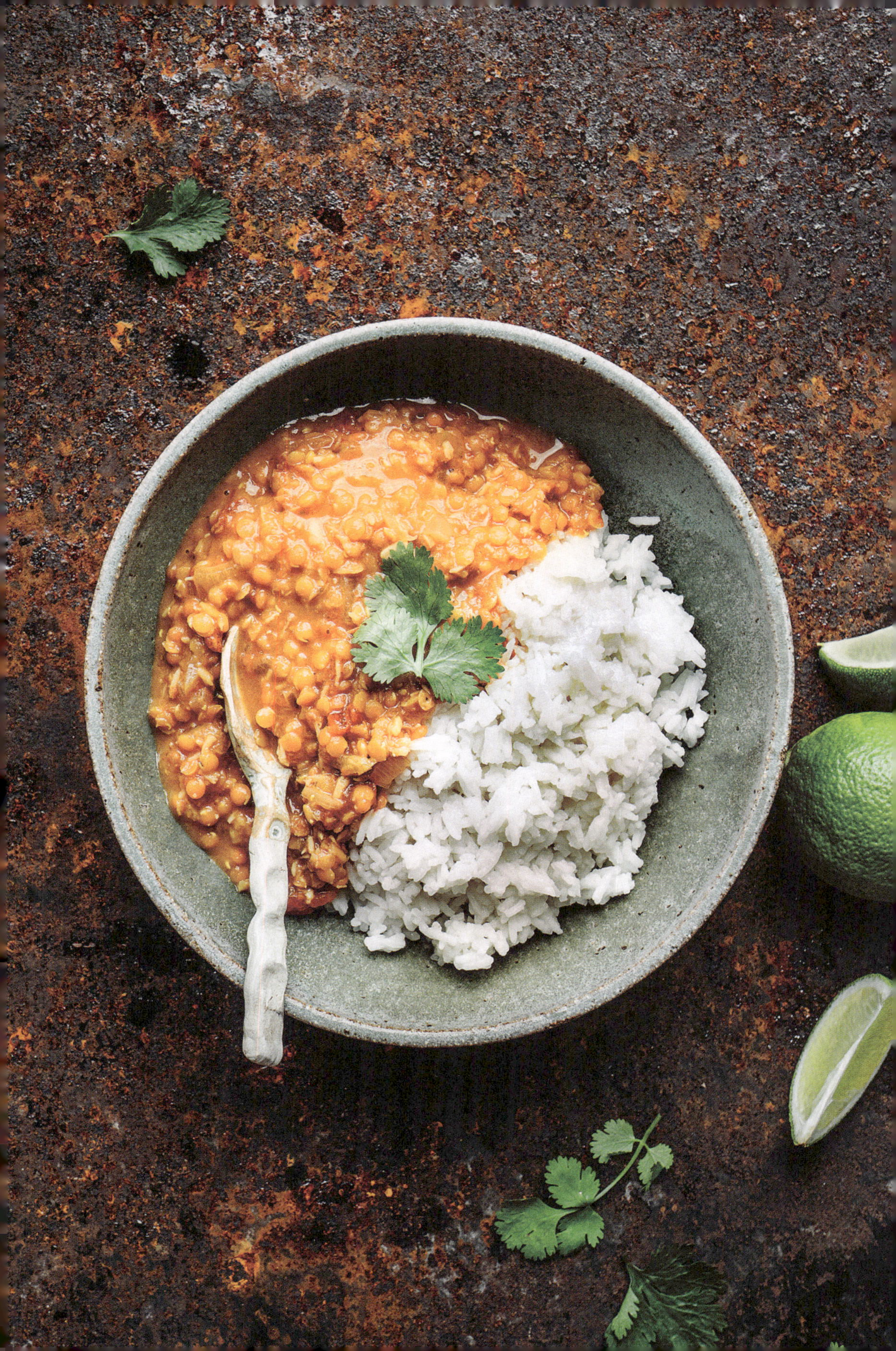

FINGER FOOD

Why eat with cutlery when your hands work just as well? This chapter looks at finger food, whether rolled, wrapped or stacked. It's probably a good idea to go and wash your hands now, because you'll definitely need them here!

RUSTIC VEGGIE BURGER

MAKES 4

FOR THE BREAD ROLLS *(makes 8)*
500 g wholemeal spelt flour
5 g fresh yeast
10 g sea salt

FOR THE BAKED POTATO WEDGES
500 g waxy potatoes
1–2 tbsp olive oil
Sea salt

FOR THE BURGERS *(makes 4)*
250 g cooked chickpeas
50 g thin-rolled porridge oats, finely ground
50 g walnuts, finely ground
150 g cooked quinoa
2 tbsp grated carrot
2 cloves garlic, crushed
1 tbsp barbecue sauce
1 tsp ground cumin
1 tsp smoked paprika
1 tsp chilli flakes
1 tsp sea salt
2–3 tbsp wholemeal spelt flour
1 tbsp rapeseed oil

EXTRAS
4 handfuls lettuce leaves
2 vine tomatoes
½ onion
2 pickled gherkins
Burger sauce (see page 120, or substitute with the sauce of your choice)
Coconut bacon (see page 116, optional)

The evening before, mix the spelt flour with the crumbled yeast and salt in a large mixing bowl. Add 325 ml of cold water and knead everything for 10 minutes to a smooth and sticky dough. Transfer the dough to a sufficiently large bowl, cover and allow to rest in the fridge overnight.

The next day, preheat the oven to 250°C. Using wet hands, tear off eight pieces of dough, each weighing about 100 g. To make each roll, gather the dough into a ball and stretch the surface several times until smooth and taut, tucking the excess underneath. To keep the surface taut, twist the excess dough at the seam using your thumb and forefinger and pinch off the protruding end. Arrange the bread rolls on a baking tray lined with baking paper with the smooth surface facing upwards and bake for 15–20 minutes. Brush them with salted water immediately after baking and allow to cool on a rack.

To make the baked potato wedges, wash and dry the potatoes thoroughly, then cut lengthways into wedges. Mix the wedges with the oil in a bowl and season with salt. Then spread them over a baking tray lined with baking paper and bake in the oven preheated to 220°C for about 30 minutes (depending on size), until golden brown, turning once after 20 minutes.

In the meantime, make the burgers. Place the chickpeas in a sieve, rinse under running water and allow to drain. Transfer to a large bowl and crush lightly with a fork to form chunks. Mix in all the remaining ingredients until combined and adjust the seasoning if necessary. Then shape the mixture into four burgers. Heat 1 tablespoon of oil in a frying pan and fry the burgers for 5 minutes on each side, until golden brown, then transfer to a container.

When ready to serve, peel or wash the remaining burger ingredients (lettuce leaves, tomatoes, onion, gherkins) and tear them into pieces or cut them into slices or rings. Slice open four rolls and stack the bottom half of each with some lettuce, a burger and sliced vegetables. Top with burger sauce and coconut bacon if desired and cover with the top half of the roll. Serve with the baked potato wedges.

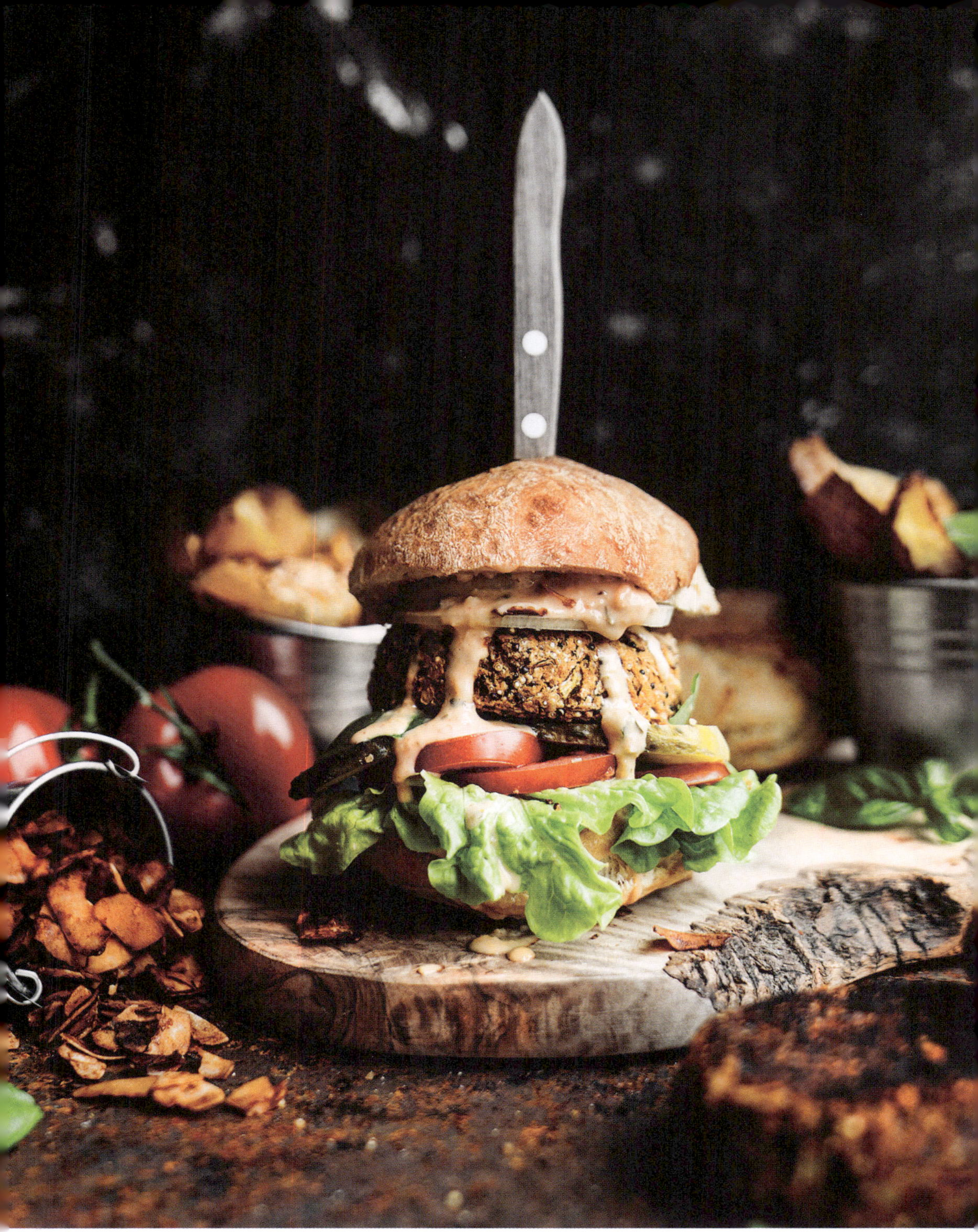

· NOTE ·

The four remaining rolls can easily be frozen – they'll always come in handy.

Alternatively, you can also make these veggie burgers using conventional burger buns (either homemade or shop-bought if you're in a hurry).

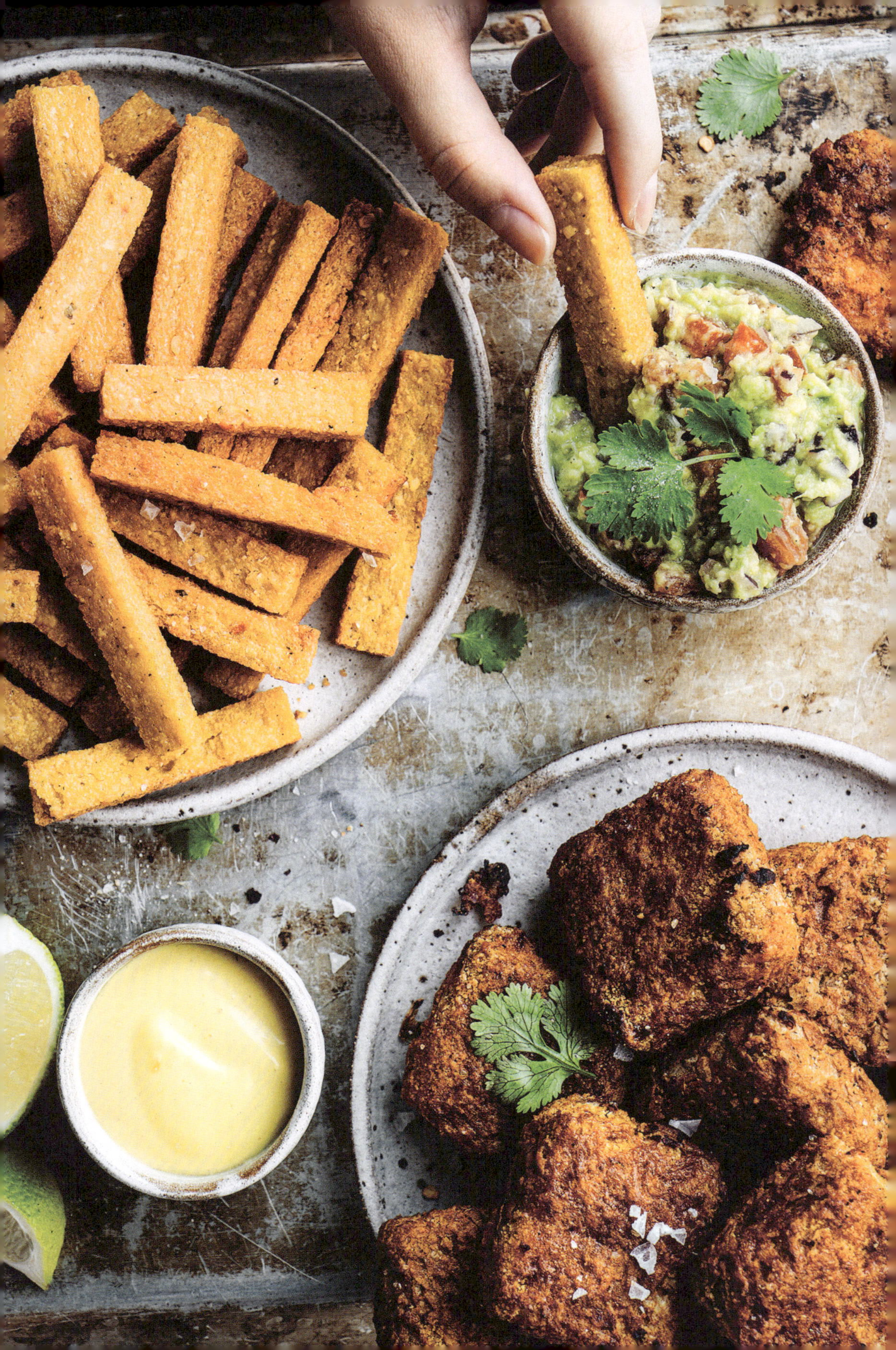

SIDE DISH DUO
FAKE FRIES & TOFU NUGGETS

FOR THE FAKE FRIES (PANISSES)
(makes 1 tray)

150 g red lentils
150 g polenta
2 tbsp yeast flakes
2 tsp vegetable stock powder
½ tsp ground turmeric
2 cloves garlic, crushed
1–2 tbsp plant-based margarine
Olive oil

Line a baking tray (approx. 25 × 30 cm) with baking paper. Finely grind the lentils in a blender, then transfer to a large pan with the polenta and all the other ingredients (except the margarine). Stir in 900 ml of water and place over the heat. Add the margarine and cook the mixture over a low-to-medium heat for 5–7 minutes, stirring constantly with a wooden spoon until it forms a firm paste that comes away from the sides of the pan. Then spread the mixture evenly on the prepared baking tray and allow to cool for 30 minutes.

In the meantime, preheat the oven to 200°C. Cut the polenta mixture into finger-length sticks. Spread them over the tray and bake for 45 minutes until crispy, turning after 25 minutes and brushing on all sides with a little olive oil. For extra crispy fries, put the tray on the top shelf for a few minutes towards the end or switch on the grill.

·ACCOMPANIMENTS·

Guacamole (see page 119)
Aïoli (see page 119)

FOR THE TOFU NUGGETS *(12 nuggets)*

400 g firm tofu
80 g cornflour
100 ml unsweetened plant-based milk
1 tbsp Thai sweet chilli sauce (shop-bought or homemade, see page 120)
80 g dry breadcrumbs
1 tbsp yeast flakes
2 tsp sweet paprika
1 tsp mild curry powder
1 tsp sea salt
½ tsp freshly ground pepper
Olive oil
BBQ sauce (optional)

Freeze the tofu overnight and thaw it out the next day. Preheat the oven to 200°C. Cut the thawed tofu into twelve equal pieces, place between kitchen paper and squeeze out the remaining liquid. Now prepare three shallow bowls for the breading process: fill the first with the cornflour, the second with the milk mixed with the sweet chilli sauce, and the last with the breadcrumbs mixed with the yeast flakes and spices. Dredge all the tofu pieces in the cornflour, then dip each one in the seasoned milk. Dredge each nugget a second time in the cornflour, dip again in the milk and, finally, roll them in the seasoned breadcrumbs. If you run out of an ingredient, refill the plates as needed.

Spread the breaded tofu nuggets over a tray lined with baking paper and bake for 30 minutes until crispy, turning after 20 minutes and brushing on all sides with a little olive oil. Brush the nuggets with BBQ sauce if desired before serving.

THE IMPOSTER SANDWICH

MAKES 1 LARGE SANDWICH

FOR THE BEAN SALAD

150 g cooked gigantes beans
1 tbsp chopped herbs (e.g. chives, parsley)
2 tsp freshly squeezed lemon juice
1 tbsp almond butter
Sea salt, freshly ground pepper

EXTRAS

1 small carrot
1 vine tomato
1 thumb-length piece of organic cucumber
½ avocado
1 tbsp freshly squeezed lemon juice
1 handful red cabbage
1 dash rice vinegar
1 handful sprouts of your choice
2 handfuls lettuce leaves
2 slices freshly baked bread

To make the bean salad, place the beans in a sieve, rinse thoroughly under running water and allow to drain. Transfer to a bowl and mash with a fork into a chunky paste, then stir in the chopped herbs, lemon juice and almond butter and season with salt and pepper.

Then prepare the other sandwich fillings. Peel the carrot and cut into thin sticks (or grate). Wash and very thinly slice the tomato and cucumber. Scoop out the flesh from the avocado, cut it into wedges and drizzle with a little lemon juice. Clean and shred the red cabbage, place in a small bowl and drizzle with the rice vinegar. Then knead it with your fingers until soft. Wash and shake dry the sprouts and lettuce leaves.

When ready to serve, cover a slice of bread with a handful of lettuce and spread the bean salad over the top. Then stack all the prepared ingredients over the bean salad as desired, top with the remaining lettuce and cover with the second slice of bread. Wrap the sandwich tightly in a sandwich bag or a piece of baking paper and cut it in half with a sharp knife before serving.

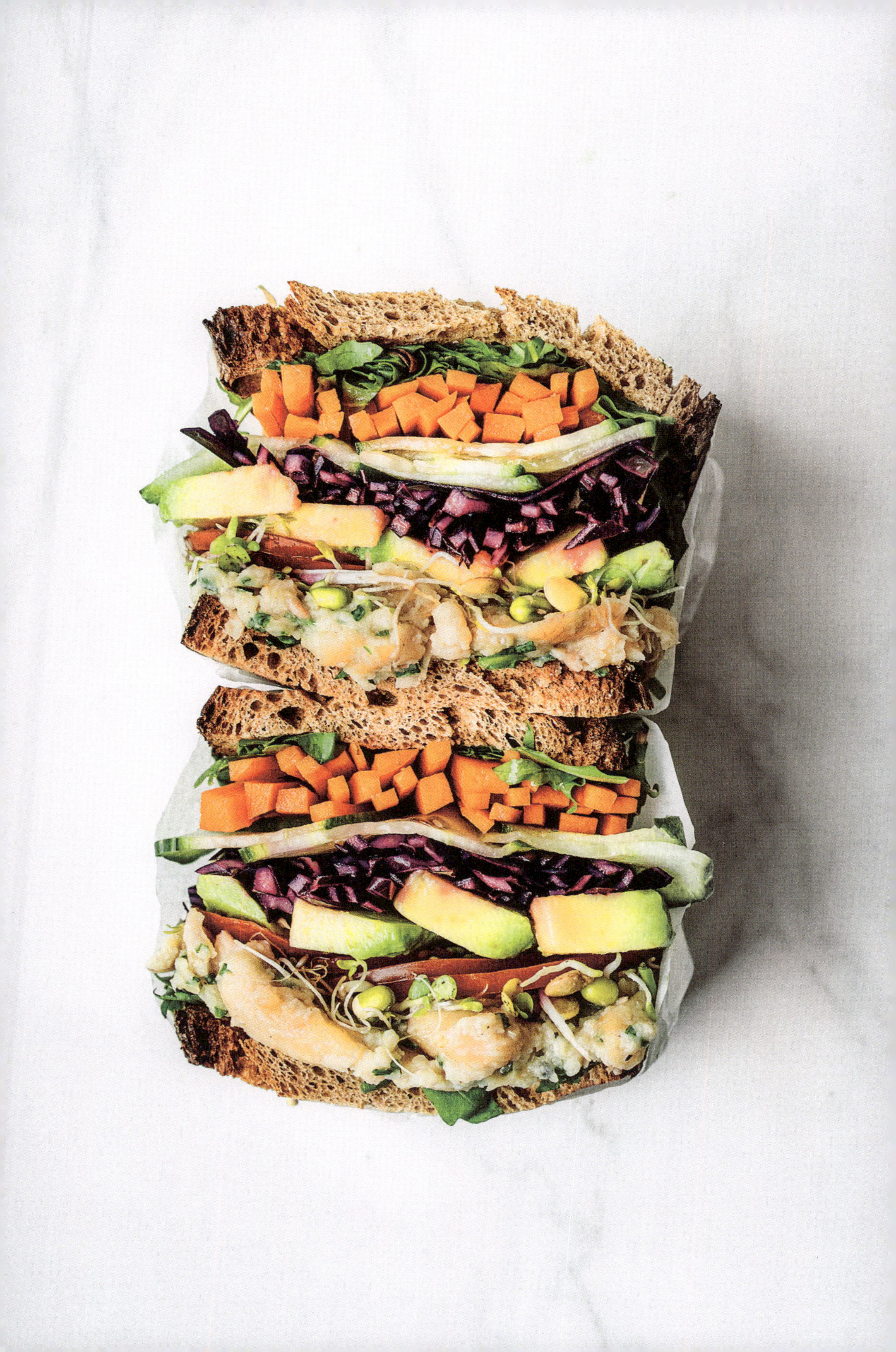

DÖNER WRAP WITH CHICKPEA PILAF

MAKES 2

FOR THE KEBAB SAUCE

200 g unsweetened soya yoghurt
1 clove garlic, crushed
1 tbsp olive oil
Sea salt

FOR THE CHICKPEA PILAF

125 g cooked chickpeas
1 tsp plant-based margarine
100 g basmati rice
Sea salt

FOR THE FILLING

1 small red onion
1 vine tomato
⅓ organic cucumber
1 tbsp chopped flat-leaf parsley
80 g red cabbage
80 g iceberg lettuce
80 g tinned sweetcorn kernels

FOR THE FLATBREADS *(makes 2)*

200 g wholemeal spelt flour, plus more for dusting
⅓ tsp sea salt

EXTRAS

Tahini sauce (see page 120, optional)

To make the kebab sauce, mix all the ingredients together in a bowl, season with salt and set aside in the fridge until ready to serve.

To make the chickpea pilaf, place the chickpeas in a sieve, rinse thoroughly under running water and allow to drain. Melt the margarine in a pan, add the rice and chickpeas and sauté until the rice turns a little translucent. Carefully add 250 ml of hot water, season with salt and bring to the boil. Cover the pan, reduce the heat to low and allow to simmer for 10–12 minutes, until the rice is cooked. Stir the mixture from time to time to keep from burning.

Prepare the other filling ingredients. Peel and finely chop the onion. Wash and halve the tomato, then cut off the stem end, de-seed and cut into small pieces. Wash and dice the cucumber. Mix everything together in a bowl with the parsley. Clean and trim the red cabbage and iceberg lettuce and cut both into very thin strips. Drain the sweetcorn in a sieve.

To make the flatbreads, mix the flour with the salt in a bowl. Mix in 100 ml of water to form a dough and knead for 10 minutes until smooth. Lightly dust the work surface with flour. Cut the dough in half and roll each half out into two very thin discs. Heat a large, dry non-stick frying pan and cook the flatbread over a medium heat for about 1 minute on each side, until it develops the bubbles characteristic of cooking in a pan.

When ready to serve, first spread kebab sauce over the centre of the warm flatbreads, then cover the sauce with the prepared vegetables and chickpea pilaf. On the side which will become the bottom end of the wrap, fold the flatbread a few centimetres over the filling (so that nothing falls out). Then roll the flatbread up tightly. Serve the wrap as is or with tahini sauce as desired.

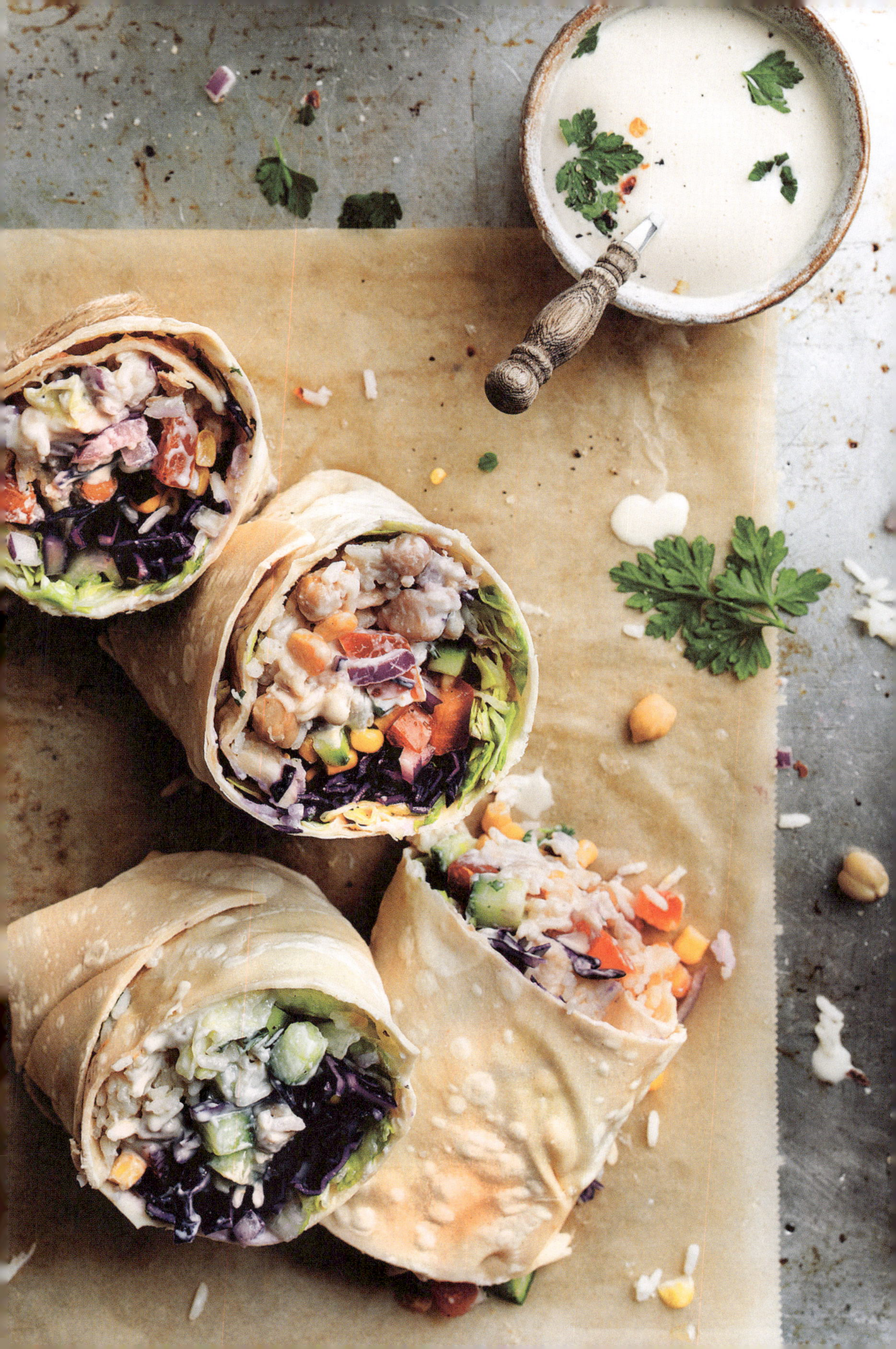

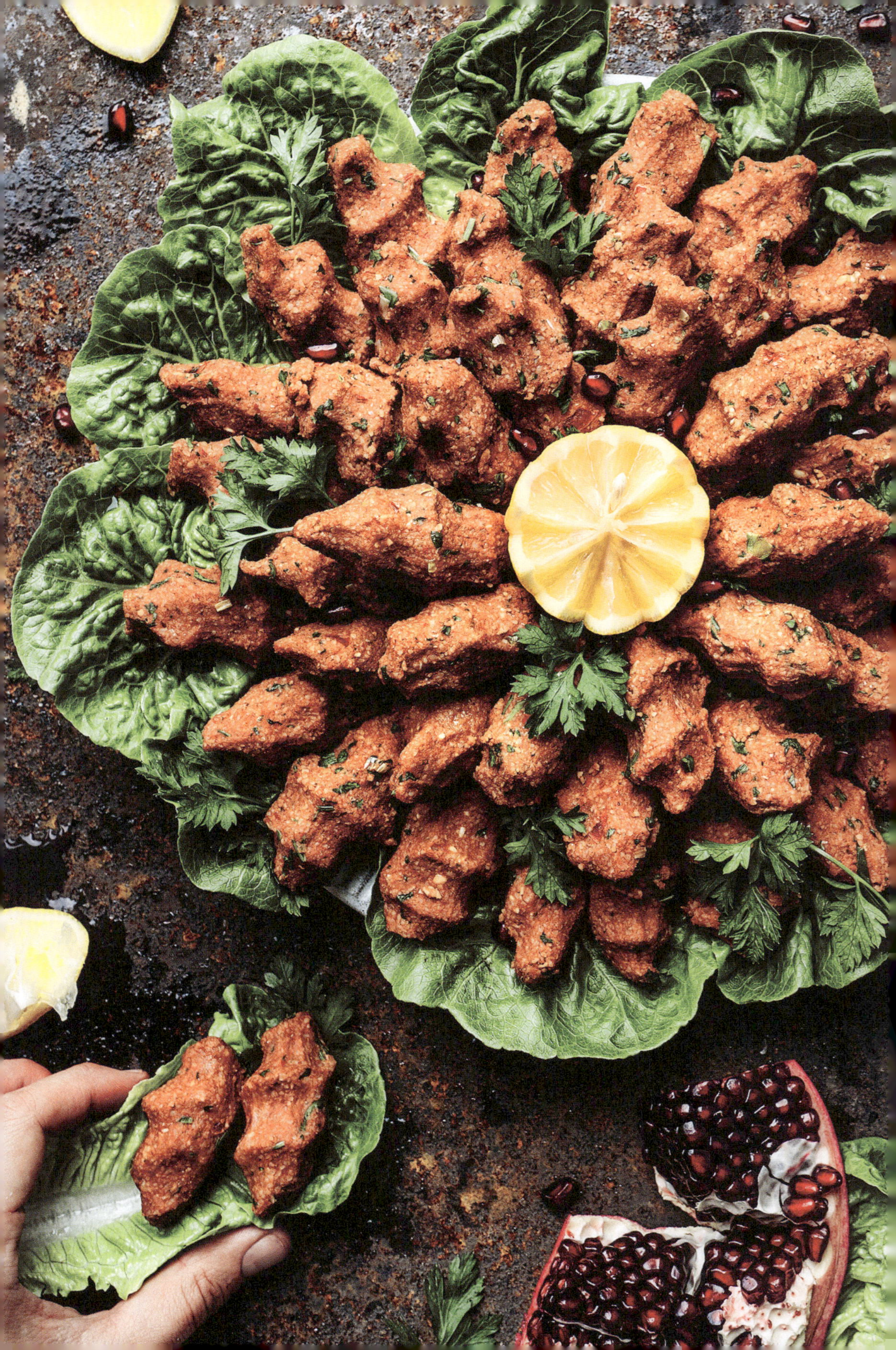

ÇIĞ KÖFTE ('RAW MEATBALLS')

SERVES 6

FOR THE KÖFTE

3 cloves garlic
5 spring onions
3 vine tomatoes
100 g shelled walnuts
500 g fine bulgur for making köfte (köftelik bulgur, available from Turkish supermarkets)
150 g hot ajvar sauce
100 g tomato purée
1 tbsp freshly squeezed lemon juice
1 tbsp agave syrup
1 tbsp chilli powder
1 tbsp sweet paprika
1 tsp ground cumin
Sea salt
½ bunch flat-leaf parsley, chopped

EXTRAS

Lettuce leaves (e.g. Cos lettuce, iceberg lettuce)
Flat-leaf parsley
Pomegranate seeds
½ lemon, decoratively cut (e.g. lemon crown)
Lemon juice

Peel and finely chop the garlic. Trim, wash and thinly slice the spring onions. Wash and halve the tomatoes, then cut off the stem end, de-seed and cut into small dice. Finely grind the walnuts in a blender.

In a large bowl, mix the bulgur with all the ingredients (except the parsley) and 150 ml of cold water, then knead with your hands for 20 minutes, until the mixture is smooth. Add a little more water if necessary. The bulgur mixture should stick and hold its shape when pressed. Season with salt and adjust the other seasonings if necessary. Finally, mix in the chopped parsley. To shape the çiğ köfte, take a walnut-sized portion of the bulgur and mould it with your fingers to create the characteristic shape.

When ready to serve, wash the lettuce and parsley and shake dry. Make a bed of lettuce leaves on a large plate, then arrange the finished çiğ köfte over them and garnish with the parsley, a few pomegranate seeds and the half lemon. Drizzle with lemon juice and serve.

VIETNAMESE SUMMER ROLLS

MAKES 8

FOR THE LEMONGRASS-FLAVOURED TOFU

200 g firm tofu
3 cloves garlic, crushed
1 stalk lemongrass, finely chopped
2 tbsp soy sauce
1 tbsp sesame oil (or substitute with olive oil)
1 tbsp rapeseed oil

FOR THE SUMMER ROLLS

60 g dried rice vermicelli noodles
2 spring onions
1 handful red cabbage
¼ organic cucumber
1 carrot
½ red pepper
1 avocado
8 Cos lettuce leaves
50 g roasted and salted peanuts
1 handful coriander
8 rice paper wrappers

EXTRAS

Peanut dip (see page 119, optional)
Thai sweet chilli sauce (shop-bought or homemade, see page 120; optional)

To make the lemongrass-flavoured tofu, drain the tofu and cut it lengthways into thin slices. Place the slices between sheets of kitchen paper and squeeze out the remaining liquid. Mix the remaining ingredients together in a bowl, then add the tofu slices, coat well and marinate in the fridge for 1 hour (or longer if desired).

To make the summer rolls, cook the rice noodles according to the packet instructions, then transfer to a sieve, refresh in cold water and allow to drain. Wash and trim the vegetables. Finely slice the spring onions, shred the red cabbage and cut the cucumber, carrot and pepper into thin sticks. Halve the avocado, remove the stone, scoop the flesh out of the shell and slice lengthways. Wash the lettuce leaves and pat dry. Finely chop the peanuts. Wash the coriander, shake dry and pluck the leaves from the stalks.

Remove the tofu slices from the marinade and fry them in a hot frying pan with 1 tablespoon of rapeseed oil on both sides until golden brown, then transfer to a container.

When ready to make the rolls, fill a large plate with cold water. One at a time, dip a rice paper wrapper into the water, allow it to drain and lay it on a second plate. Place a little coriander in the centre first, then add a lettuce leaf and top with rice noodles, tofu and vegetables. Sprinkle with chopped peanuts. Fold the side of the wrapper closest to you over the filling, then fold in the sides and roll up the wrapper tightly.

Arrange the summer rolls on a large plate and serve together with the peanut dip and sweet chilli sauce or another sauce of your choice.

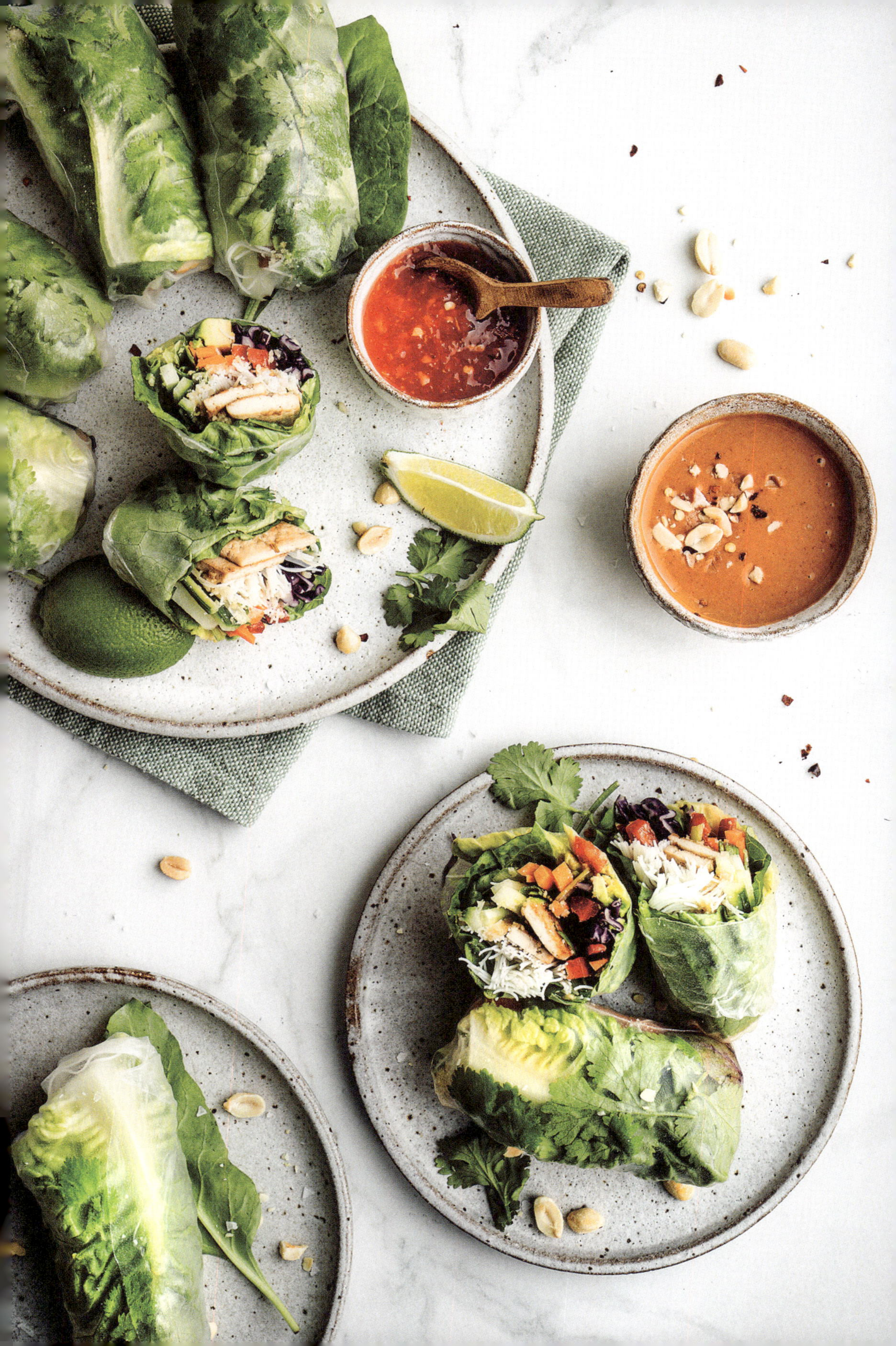

SWEET TREATS

Who says that 'sweet' and 'healthy' are opposites? Mother Nature gives us a wide variety of delicious foods that combine both. There's something here not only for young and old alike, but also for health-conscious sweet tooths.

PEANUT CARAMEL BARS

MAKES 12

FOR THE BARS
100 g thin-rolled porridge oats
50 g + 100 g roasted and salted peanuts
250 g pitted dates (preferably soft, e.g. Medjool)
50 g peanut butter

FOR THE CHOCOLATE COATING
150 g dark chocolate
1 tbsp coconut oil

Finely grind the oats together with 50 g of peanuts in a blender and transfer to a bowl. Coarsely chop the remaining 100 g of peanuts and transfer to a second bowl. In a blender, blend the dates with the peanut butter and 3 tablespoons of water to a smooth paste.

For the caramel layer, mix 200 g of the date mixture from the blender into the coarsely chopped peanuts.

For the base layer, add the oat and peanut mixture to the remaining date mixture in the blender and blend until a dough forms. Transfer the dough to a bowl and knead briefly with your hands, then place it on a sheet of baking paper and press into a rectangular strip (approx. 30 × 6 cm). Spread the caramel over the dough and smooth the surface using moistened fingers. Transfer to the freezer for 30 minutes, then wet the blade of a knife and cut out finger-thick bars. Freeze again for 1 hour.

For the chocolate coating, coarsely chop the dark chocolate and melt it in a bowl over hot water, then stir in the coconut oil.
Coat the frozen bars with the melted chocolate, then store them in an airtight container in the fridge or freezer.

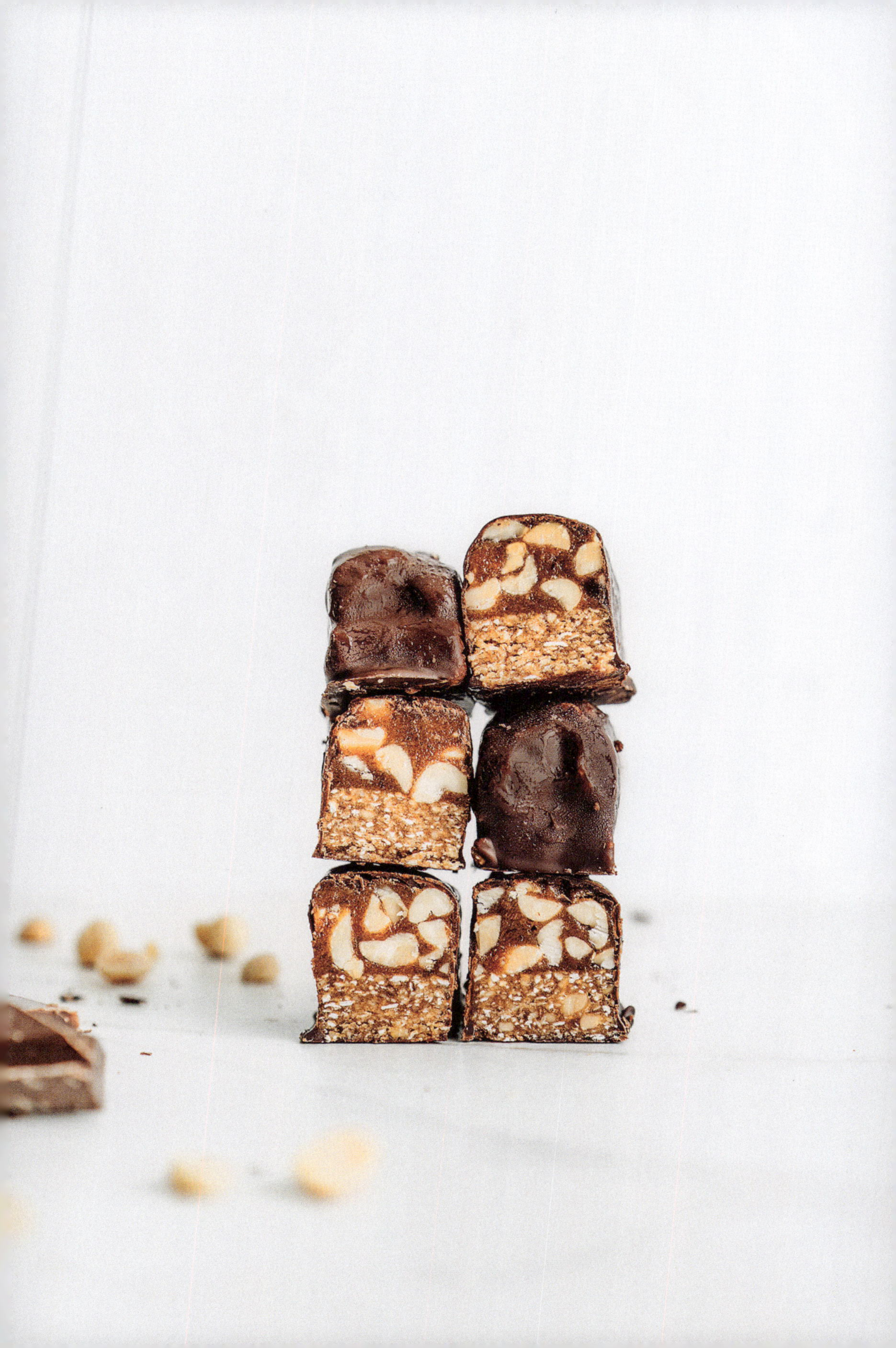

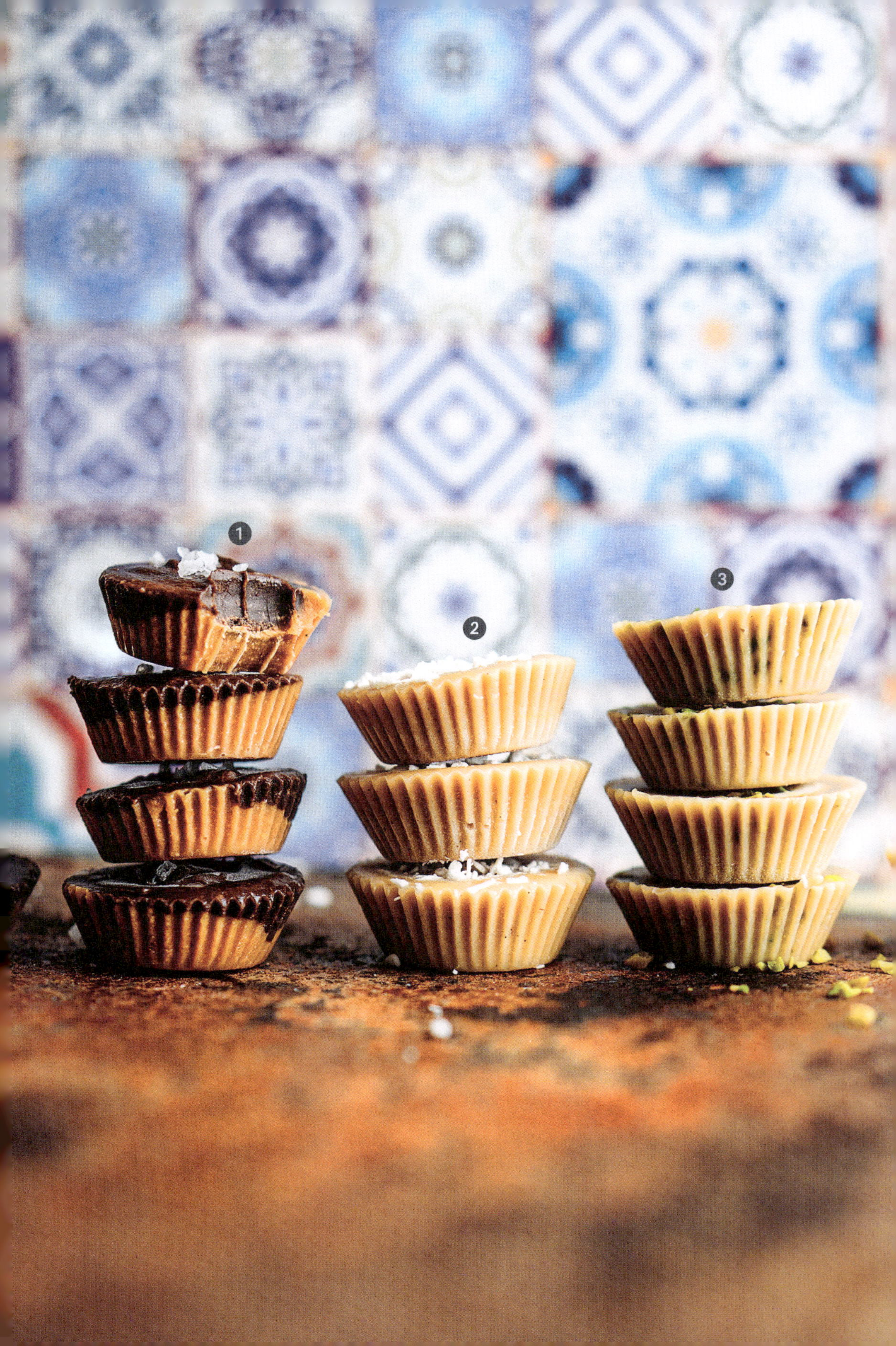
1
2
3

FREEZER FUDGE

3 VERSIONS - SERVES 8

❶ PEANUT BUTTER FREEZER FUDGE

100 g peanut butter
2 tbsp maple syrup
2 tbsp coconut oil, melted
2 tbsp cocoa powder
Sea salt flakes

In a bowl, mix the peanut butter with the maple syrup and coconut oil. Line a small muffin tin with eight paper cases and divide half of the mixture evenly between them. Add the cocoa to the remaining mixture in the bowl and mix until combined, then pour an even amount over the mixture already inside the muffin cases. Swirl a cocktail stick through both mixtures to create a marble effect and then sprinkle with salt flakes. Freeze until the fudge is firm (about 1 hour). Then remove the fudge from the paper cases and store in an airtight container in the freezer.

❷ RAFFAELO FREEZER FUDGE

100 g white almond butter
2 tbsp maple syrup
2 tbsp coconut oil, melted
½ tsp vanilla extract
Desiccated coconut

In a bowl, mix the almond butter with the maple syrup, coconut oil and vanilla extract. Line a small muffin tin with eight paper cases and divide the mixture evenly between them. Sprinkle with desiccated coconut and freeze until the fudge is firm (about 1 hour). Then remove the fudge from the paper cases and store in an airtight container in the freezer.

❸ HALVA FREEZER FUDGE

100 g tahini (sesame paste)
2 tbsp maple syrup
2 tbsp coconut oil, melted
1 tbsp chopped pistachio nuts

Mix all the ingredients together in a bowl. Line a small muffin tin with eight paper cases and divide the mixture evenly between them. Freeze until the fudge is firm (about 1 hour). Then remove the fudge from the paper cases and store in an airtight container in the freezer.

• NOTE •

Instead of using muffin tins, you can make these fudge recipes using tartlet moulds or ramekins placed on a stable surface that can go into the freezer. Alternatively, you can also use large muffin cases, in which case there should be enough of the mixture to fill five. Important: As this fudge melts at room temperature, remember to only take it out of the freezer immediately before eating.

BLISS BALLS

6 VERSIONS

1 WALNUT BROWNIE
100 g pitted dates
60 g shelled walnuts
30 g thin-rolled porridge oats
1 tbsp cocoa powder
1 pinch of sea salt
30 g chopped dark chocolate (optional)

2 HAZELNUT & CINNAMON
100 g pitted dates
100 g hazelnuts
20 g thin-rolled porridge oats
1 tbsp ground cinnamon
1 pinch of ground cloves
1 pinch of sea salt

3 SALTED PEANUT
100 g pitted dates
100 g roasted and salted peanuts
20 g thin-rolled porridge oats
1 pinch of sea salt

4 CHIA SEED & LEMON CAKE
80 g pitted dates
80 g cashew nuts
30 g thin-rolled porridge oats
1 tbsp freshly squeezed lemon juice
1 tbsp chia seeds
1 tsp untreated lemon zest

5 GOLDEN MILK
100 g pitted dates
60 g desiccated coconut
40 g thin-rolled porridge oats
30 g cashew nuts
10 g freshly grated ginger
1 tsp ground turmeric
1 pinch of freshly ground pepper
1 pinch of sea salt

6 STRAWBERRY & VANILLA
100 g pitted dates
80 g cashew nuts
20 g desiccated coconut
10 g freeze-dried strawberries
½ tsp vanilla extract

· METHOD ·

Put all the ingredients into a blender and blend until the mixture has the consistency of wet sand. Transfer the mixture to a bowl and knead by hand to a dough. Then divide the mixture into eight portions and shape them into balls by pressing firmly with your fingers and then rolling between the palms of your hands while applying light pressure. Store the bliss balls in an airtight container in the fridge or freezer.

· NOTE ·

The consistency of the bliss balls can vary depending on the ingredients and the blending step. If the dough is too crumbly or firm, add more wet ingredients (e.g. a little nut butter, maple syrup or water). If the bliss balls are too soft, ground nuts or porridge oats can help make them firmer.

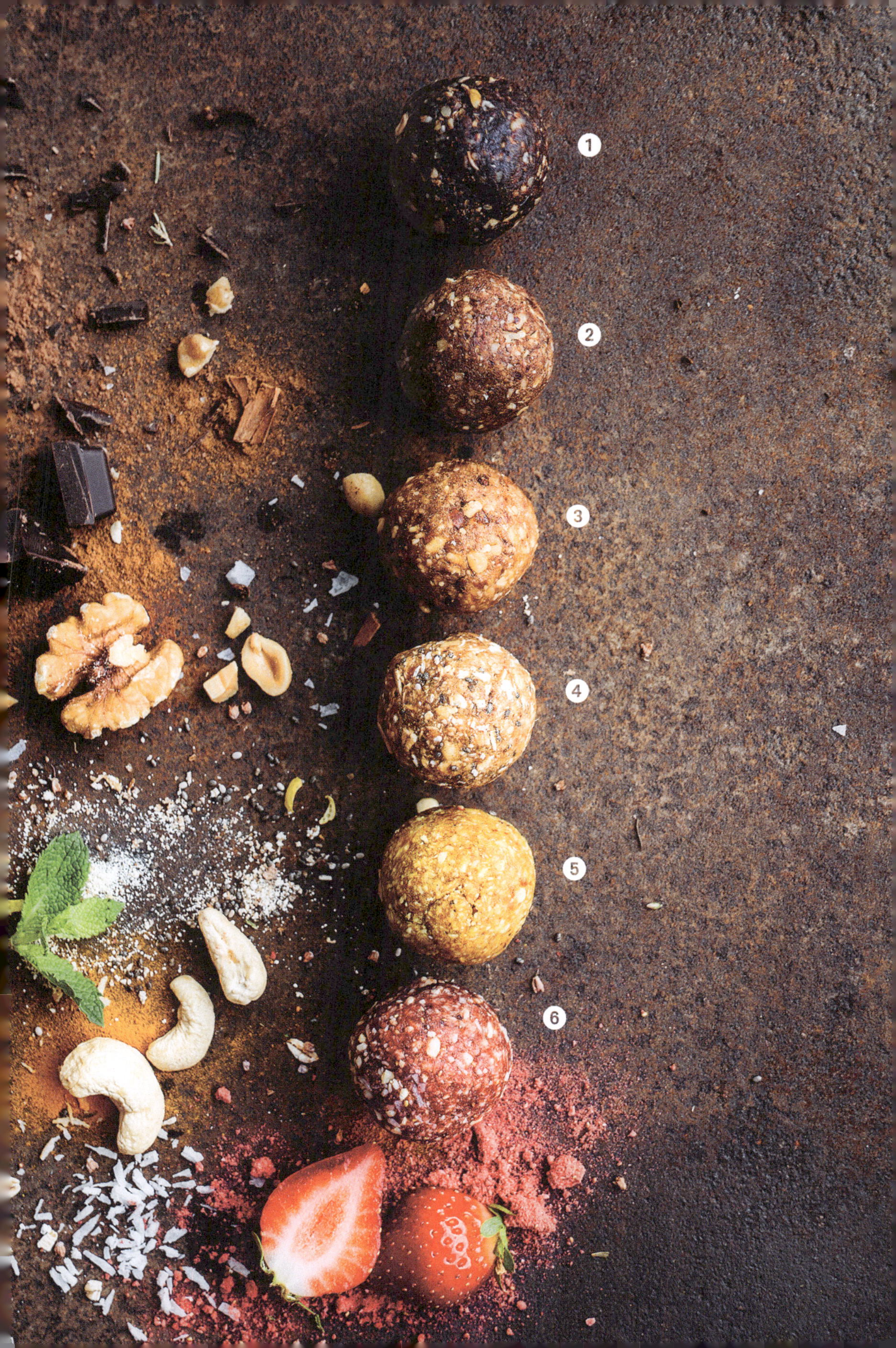
1
2
3
4
5
6

BLACK BEAN BROWNIES

MAKES 16 SMALL BROWNIES

250 g cooked black beans
120 g peanut butter
100 g agave syrup
20 g cocoa powder
¼ tsp sea salt
50 g dark chocolate

Preheat the oven to 180°C.

Place the beans in a sieve, rinse thoroughly under running water and allow to drain. Then transfer to a blender together with the peanut butter and agave syrup and blend until smooth. Add the cocoa powder and salt and blend again until combined. Chop the chocolate into chunks and fold them into the mixture.

Transfer the brownie mixture to a baking tray lined with baking paper and spread it out into a 2.5-cm-thick square. Bake for 20–25 minutes. Then remove the brownie from the oven, allow to cool for 20 minutes and cut it into 16 squares.

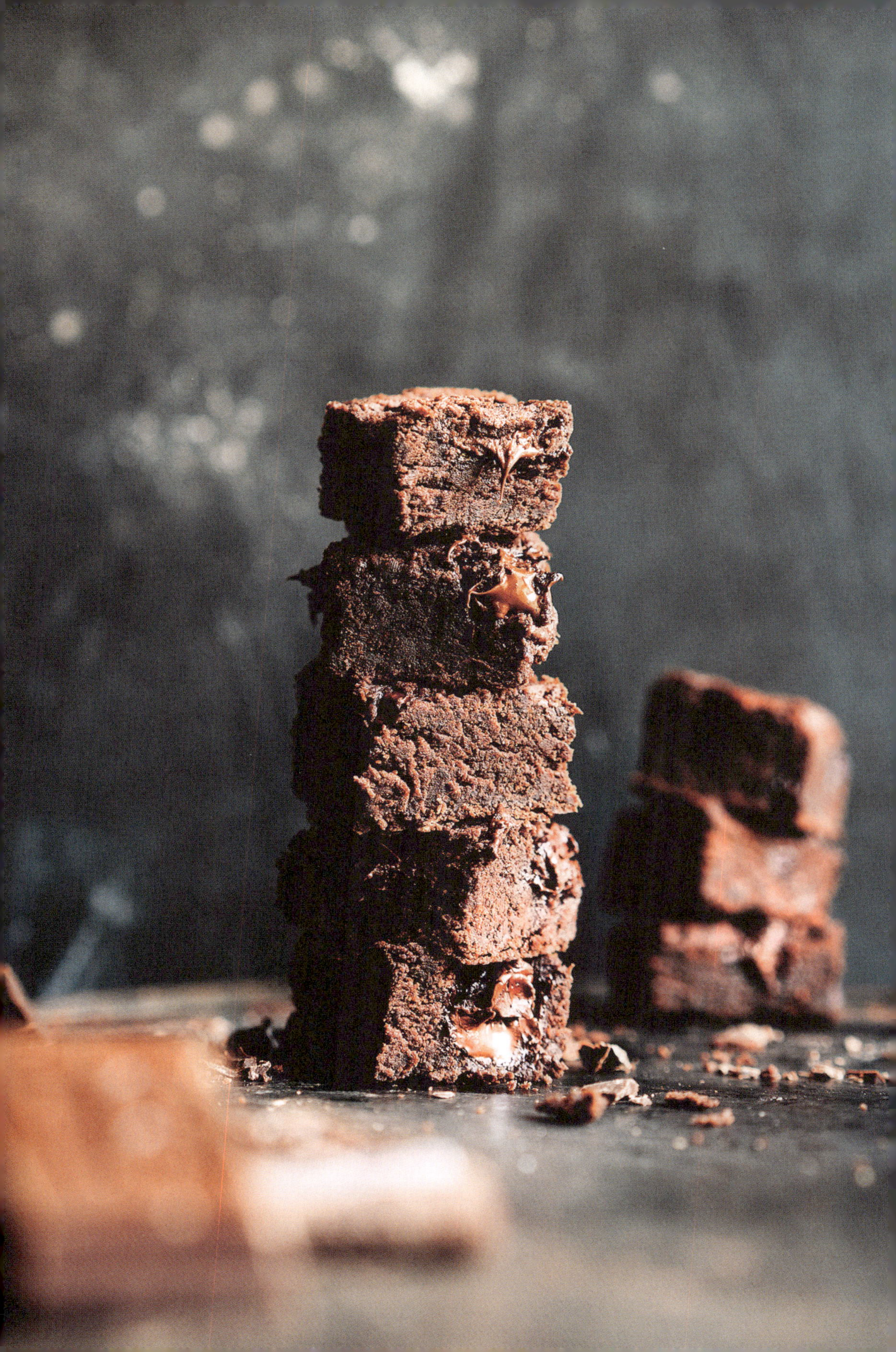

FUNFETTI COOKIE DOUGH

SERVES 2

FOR THE EDIBLE COOKIE DOUGH

250 g cooked chickpeas
70 g pitted dates (preferably soft, e.g. Medjool)
30 g almond butter
50 ml plant-based milk
40 g ground almonds
30 g thin-rolled porridge oats, finely ground
1 tsp vanilla extract
1 pinch of sea salt

EXTRAS

2 tbsp sugar decorations (e.g. Smarties, hundreds and thousands)
Fruit for dipping (e.g. apple and pear slices)

Place the chickpeas in a sieve, rinse thoroughly under running water and allow to drain. Then transfer to a blender together with the dates, almond butter and plant-based milk and blend to a smooth paste. Then add the almonds, oats, vanilla extract and salt and blend until combined.

This cookie dough is best chilled before serving, although it can be eaten directly. When ready to serve, divide the cookie dough between two bowls, sprinkle over with your sugar decoration of choice and accompany with the fruit of your choice.

THE PERFECT EDIBLE COOKIE DOUGH

1 Essentials: The best chickpeas to use are the ones you cook yourself at home because they have a flourier texture and less of a chickpea flavour than tinned chickpeas. Adding baking soda to the cooking water (1 teaspoon to 1 litre of water) speeds up the cooking process, and the chickpeas soften more quickly and become more delicate and easier to blend.

2 Counteracting: Even if you love chickpeas, tasting them in cookie dough can be off-putting. To tone their flavour down as much as possible, it's important to use other ingredients to counteract it. In this case, for example, dates are more suitable for sweetening than agave syrup. In general, if the cookie dough tastes too strongly of chickpeas, it means that there aren't enough other ingredients in the dough. More oats, almonds or dates will help with this. Ultimately, the ratio of ingredients is a matter of taste. As fat is a good flavour carrier, 1 tablespoon of nut butter can work wonders.

3 Order: It's important that all ingredients are chopped up as finely as possible. For this reason, the order in which the ingredients are used is crucial.
Start by preparing the dry ingredients (finely grind in a blender and set aside), then blend the wet ingredients until smooth. Only mix the two together at the end and blend to combine. If the dates aren't soft enough, simply pour hot water over them and soak them for 10 minutes, then drain them and squeeze out the remaining liquid.

4 Blender: The better the blender, the easier blending becomes and the better the result. However, this doesn't mean that you actually need a high-performance blender to make delicious cookie dough. If the chickpeas and dates are soft enough and the order of blending is followed, everything should go smoothly.

5 Patience: The blender is your friend, not your enemy. If you give it enough attention, it will do just about anything for you, like making the perfect cookie dough.

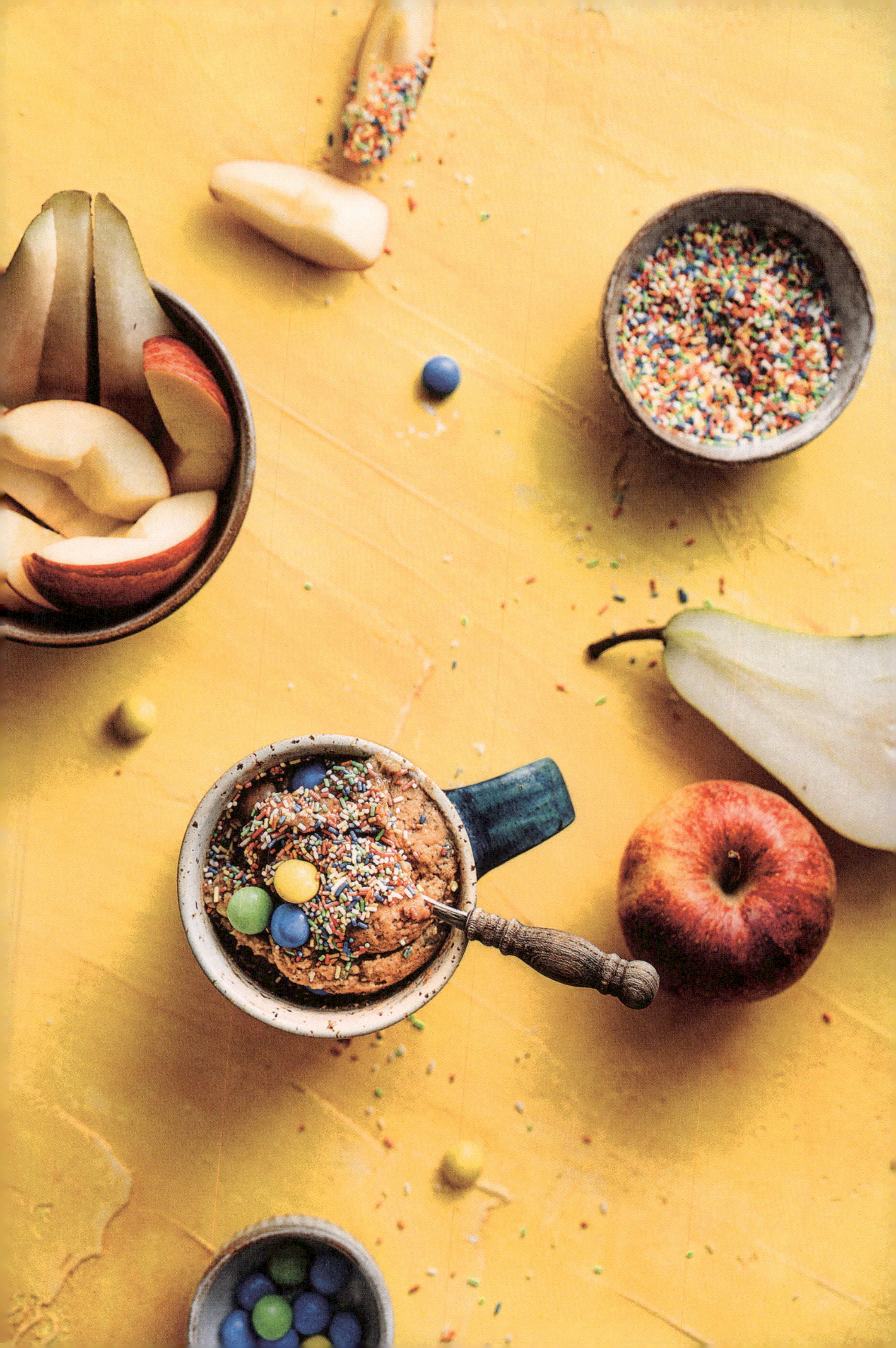

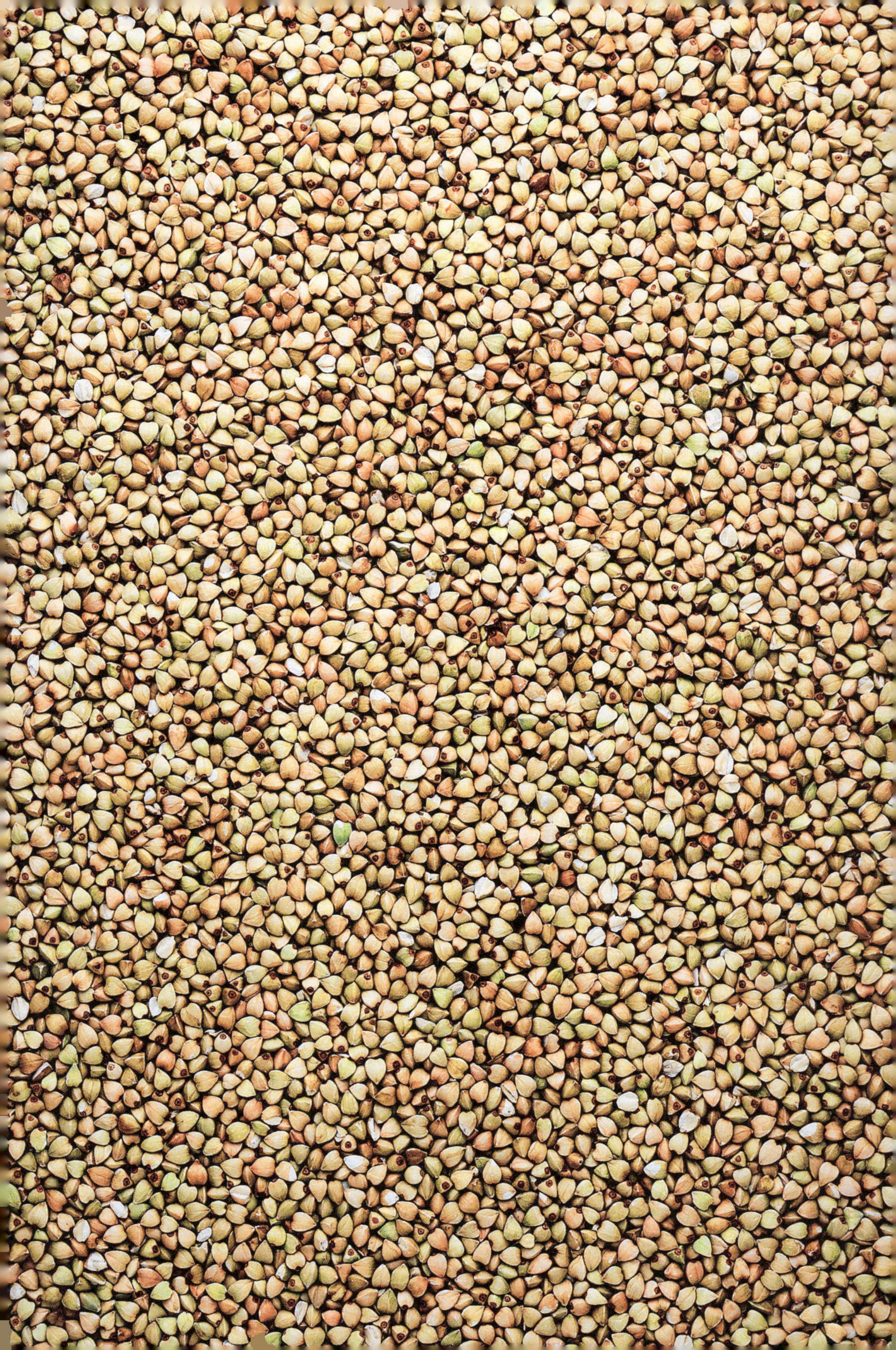

HOMEMADE

Peanut dip and Thai sweet chilli sauce make the perfect accompaniment for Asian dishes, while a bowl inspired by the Middle East tastes particularly delicious with a dollop of hummus. What about Mexican? In that case, you'll want a freshly made guacamole or a nacho cheese dip to round it off. Toppings bring out the best in bowl food – not only with their flavours but also with the additional nutrients they provide. Browse this chapter and find out what you like best.

TO TOP IT ALL OFF

6 BRILLIANT TOPPINGS

1 GOMASHIO (JAPANESE SESAME SALT
(makes about 250 g)

250 g sesame seeds
1 tbsp coarse sea salt

Toast the sesame seeds in a dry non-stick pan over a low heat until the seeds become fragrant and start popping. Add the salt and toast briefly together, then transfer the mixture into a bowl and allow to cool completely. Grind in a mortar or blender to a medium-fine texture.

2 PLAINTAIN CHIPS *(makes 2 portions)*

2 ripe green plantains
1 tbsp coconut oil, melted
Sea salt

Preheat the oven to 175°C (fan).
Peel and very thinly slice the plantains, preferably using a mandoline. Transfer to a bowl and carefully mix with the oil. Then spread the slices over a baking tray lined with baking paper and sprinkle with a little sea salt. Bake for 20 minutes, until golden brown. Remove the plantain chips from the oven and allow to cool completely.

3 CASHEW PARMESAN *(makes about 120 g)*

100 g cashew nuts
20 g yeast flakes
½ tsp garlic powder
½ tsp sea salt
1 pinch of ground turmeric

Put all the ingredients into a blender and grind to a fine and even powder.

4 QUINOA CRUNCH *(makes 1 tray)*

100 g cooked quinoa
50 g pumpkin seeds
50 g sunflower seeds
50 g buckwheat
1 tbsp hot curry powder
1 tbsp agave syrup
1 tbsp soy sauce
1 tbsp olive oil
Sea salt

Preheat the oven to 180°C. Mix all the ingredients together in a bowl. Spread the mixture over a baking tray lined with baking paper and bake for about 20 minutes, turning everything over after 10 minutes. Remove the quinoa crunch from the oven and allow to cool completely.

5 COCONUT BACON *(makes 1 tray)*

2 tbsp soy sauce
1–2 tbsp agave syrup
1 tbsp liquid smoke
1 tsp smoked paprika (optional)
1 tsp olive oil
130 g coconut chips

Preheat the oven to 160°C. Mix all the ingredients (except the coconut chips) together in a large bowl. Then mix in the coconut chips. Spread the mixture evenly over a baking tray lined with baking paper and bake for 10 minutes, then turn everything over and bake for a further 5–7 minutes (watch closely in the final minutes to keep from burning). Remove the coconut bacon from the oven and allow to cool completely.

6 ROASTED CHICKPEAS *(makes 2 portions)*

250 g cooked chickpeas
2 tsp olive oil
½ tsp sweet paprika
½ tsp ground cumin
Sea salt

Preheat the oven to 200°C. Place the chickpeas in a sieve, rinse under running water and allow to drain. Then transfer to a clean cloth and gently pat dry, removing any loose skins. Transfer to a bowl and mix in the oil, then add the spices and mix everything together. Spread the seasoned chickpeas over a baking tray lined with baking paper and roast for about 30 minutes, until golden brown, turning occasionally. Remove the roasted chickpeas from the oven and allow to cool completely.

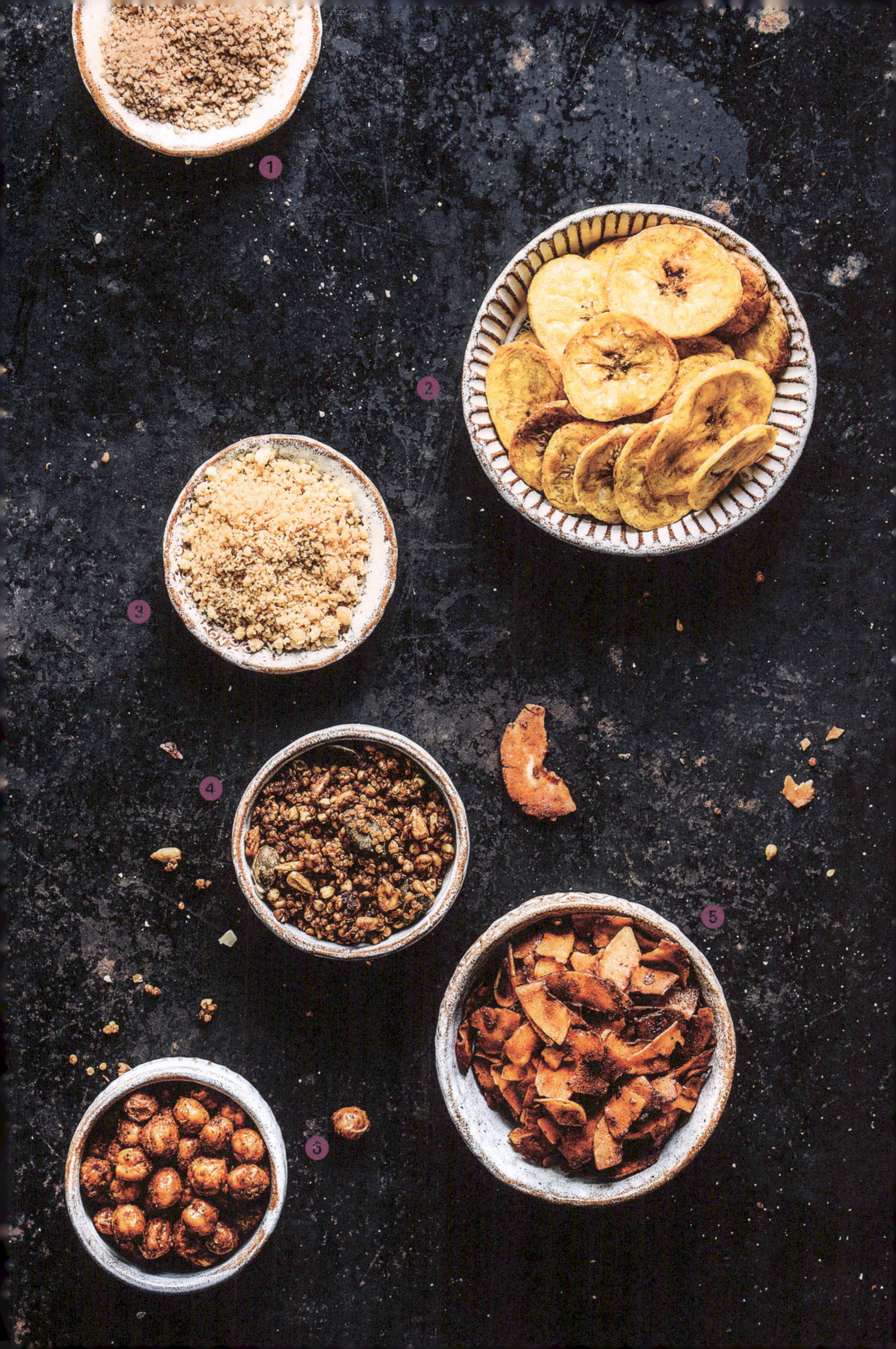
1
2
3
4
5
6

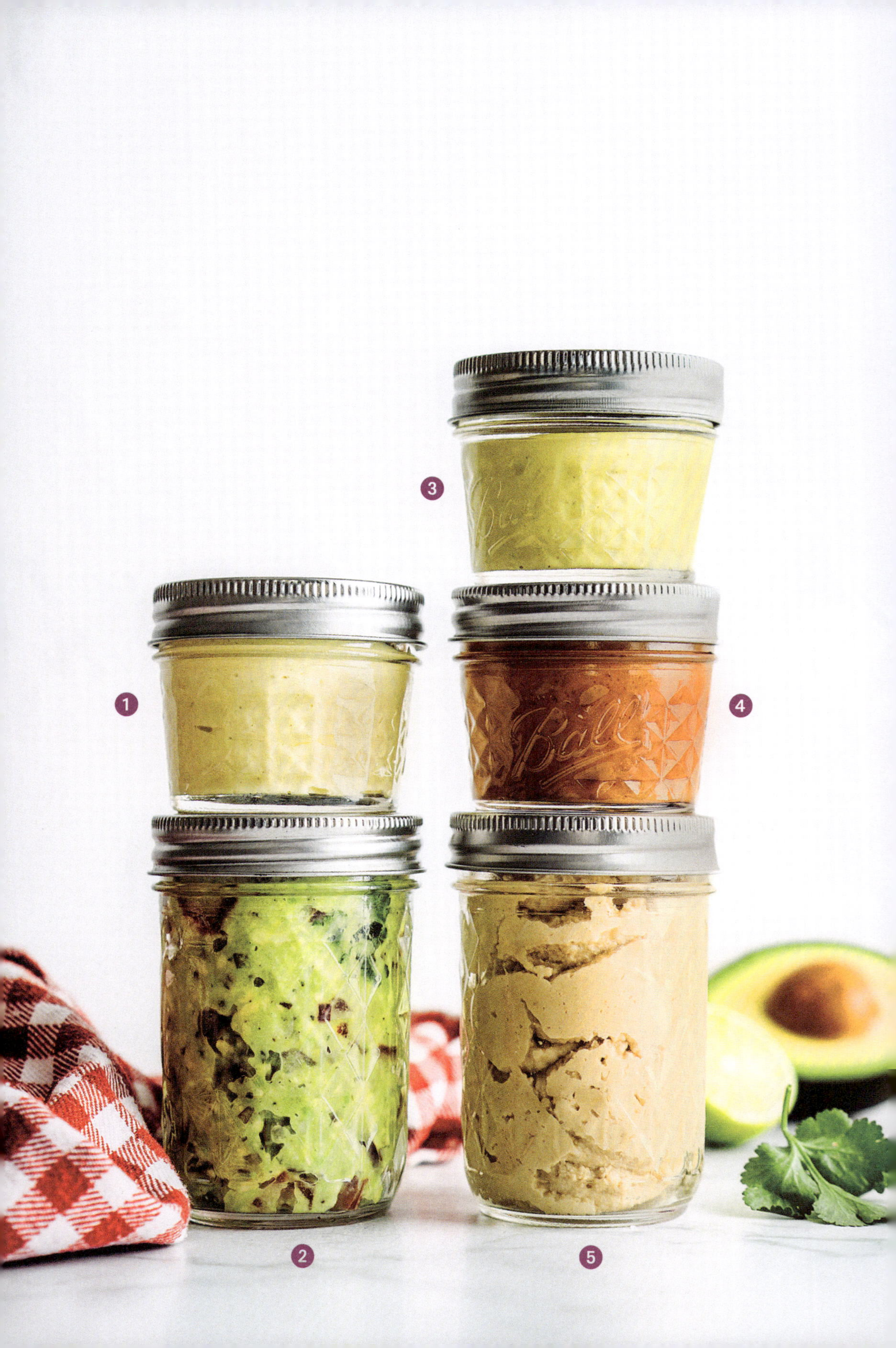
3
1
4
Ball
2
5

TIME FOR A DIP?

5 DIPS FOR EVERY OCCASION

1 AÏOLI *(makes about 150 ml)*

50 ml unsweetened soya milk, at room temperature
1 clove garlic, chopped
1 tsp apple cider vinegar
100 ml rapeseed oil
½ tsp medium hot mustard
Sea salt

Put the soya milk, garlic and vinegar into a mixing beaker and blend until frothy using a stick blender. Add the oil in a thin stream while blending to a thick emulsion. Season with the mustard and salt, transfer to a screw-top jar and chill before serving.

2 GUACAMOLE *(makes 2 portions)*

½ red onion
1 small clove garlic
½ vine tomato
1 ripe avocado
Juice of ½ lime
Sea salt, freshly ground pepper

Peel and very finely chop the onion and garlic. Wash, de-seed and finely dice the tomato. Halve the avocado, remove the stone and scoop out the flesh. Put the avocado into a bowl and mash with a fork, then add all the ingredients and mix until combined. Season with salt and pepper and serve as fresh as possible.

3 NACHO CHEESE DIP *(makes about 350 ml)*

200 g floury potatoes (peeled before weighing)
1 small onion
½ carrot
50 g cashew nuts
15 g yeast flakes
1 tsp medium hot mustard
2 pickled jalapeño chilli slices + 1 tbsp of the pickling liquid
Sea salt, freshly grated nutmeg

Peel the potatoes, onion and carrot and cut into small dice. Put the vegetables and cashews into a pan of lightly salted water and cook until soft. Then drain in a sieve, collecting the cooking liquid, and refresh briefly in cold water. Transfer the vegetables and cashews to a blender, add all the other ingredients and 50 ml of the cooking liquid and blend to the consistency of a smooth sauce. Add a little more water if necessary. Season the dip with salt and nutmeg and serve warm.

4 PEANUT DIP *(makes 2 portions)*

50 g peanut butter
1 tbsp soy sauce
½ tbsp agave syrup
½ tbsp freshly squeezed lime juice
2 tsp sriracha (hot chilli sauce, optional)

Mix all the ingredients with 3 tablespoons of water in a small bowl. Adjust the amount of liquid as needed.

5 HUMMUS *(makes about 400 ml)*

125 g dried chickpeas, soaked for 12–24 hours (or use 300 g cooked chickpeas)
½ tsp bicarbonate of soda
1–2 cloves garlic, chopped
Juice of 1 lemon
1 tsp ground cumin
½ tsp sea salt
80 g tahini (sesame paste)
3 ice cubes

Place the soaked chickpeas in a sieve, rinse thoroughly under running water and allow to drain. Transfer to a saucepan, add the baking soda and 800 ml water and cook for 30–45 minutes until very soft. Transfer to a sieve and refresh in cold water. Put the garlic, lemon juice, cumin and salt into a blender and blend, then add the chickpeas, tahini and ice cubes. Blend everything to a smooth and creamy paste.

DON'T FORGET THE SAUCE!

4 SAUCES TO FALL IN LOVE WITH

1 CHIPOTLE SAUCE *(makes about 240 ml)*

80 g cashew nuts, soaked for 4 hours or overnight
1 chipotle in adobo sauce (dried, smoked and pickled jalapeño chilli; available online)
1 clove garlic, chopped
1–2 tbsp freshly squeezed lime juice
1 tsp agave syrup
1/2 tsp smoked paprika
Sea salt

Drain the soaked cashews in a sieve, then transfer to a blender with 100 ml water and the remaining ingredients and blend until smooth. Adjust the amount of liquid as required and season the sauce with salt.

2 THAI SWEET CHILLI SAUCE *(makes about 400 ml)*

1/2 red pepper
2 Thai chilli peppers (available from Asian supermarkets)
4 cloves garlic
125 ml rice vinegar
125 g sugar
1 tbsp cornflour
1 tbsp finely grated carrot (optional)
1 tsp sea salt

Clean and trim the pepper and chillies, peel the garlic and cut everything into small pieces. Put the pepper, chillies and garlic into a mixing beaker, add the vinegar and 125 ml of water and finely chop everything using a stick blender. Transfer the mixture to a pan, add the sugar and bring to the boil. Reduce the heat to low and simmer for 3 minutes while stirring until the sugar has completely dissolved. Make a slurry by mixing the cornflour with 2 tablespoons of water and stir it into the sauce, together with the grated carrot and salt. Allow to simmer stirring constantly, until the sauce thickens. Transfer the sauce to a screw-top jar and allow to cool. This sauce should be stored in the fridge and will keep for a good 2 months.

3 TAHINI SAUCE *(makes about 160 ml)*

80 g tahini (sesame paste)
2 tbsp freshly squeezed lemon juice
1 clove garlic, crushed
1 pinch of ground cumin
1 pinch of cayenne pepper
Sea salt

Place the tahini, lemon juice, and garlic in a bowl. Slowly stir in enough water until the sauce reaches the desired consistency (about 80 ml). Then season to taste with the spices and salt.

4 BURGER SAUCE *(makes about 275 ml)*

80 g cashew nuts, soaked for 4 hours or overnight
1 clove garlic, chopped
3 tbsp tomato ketchup
2 tsp sriracha (hot chilli sauce, optional)
2 tsp medium hot mustard
2 tbsp finely chopped pickled gherkin + 1 tbsp of pickling liquid
1 tbsp finely chopped onion
Sea salt

Drain the soaked cashew nuts in a sieve and transfer to a blender. Add 100 ml of water, the garlic, ketchup, sriracha and mustard and blend until smooth. Then gently mix in the pickled gherkin, pickling liquid and onion. Adjust the amount of liquid as required and season the sauce with salt.

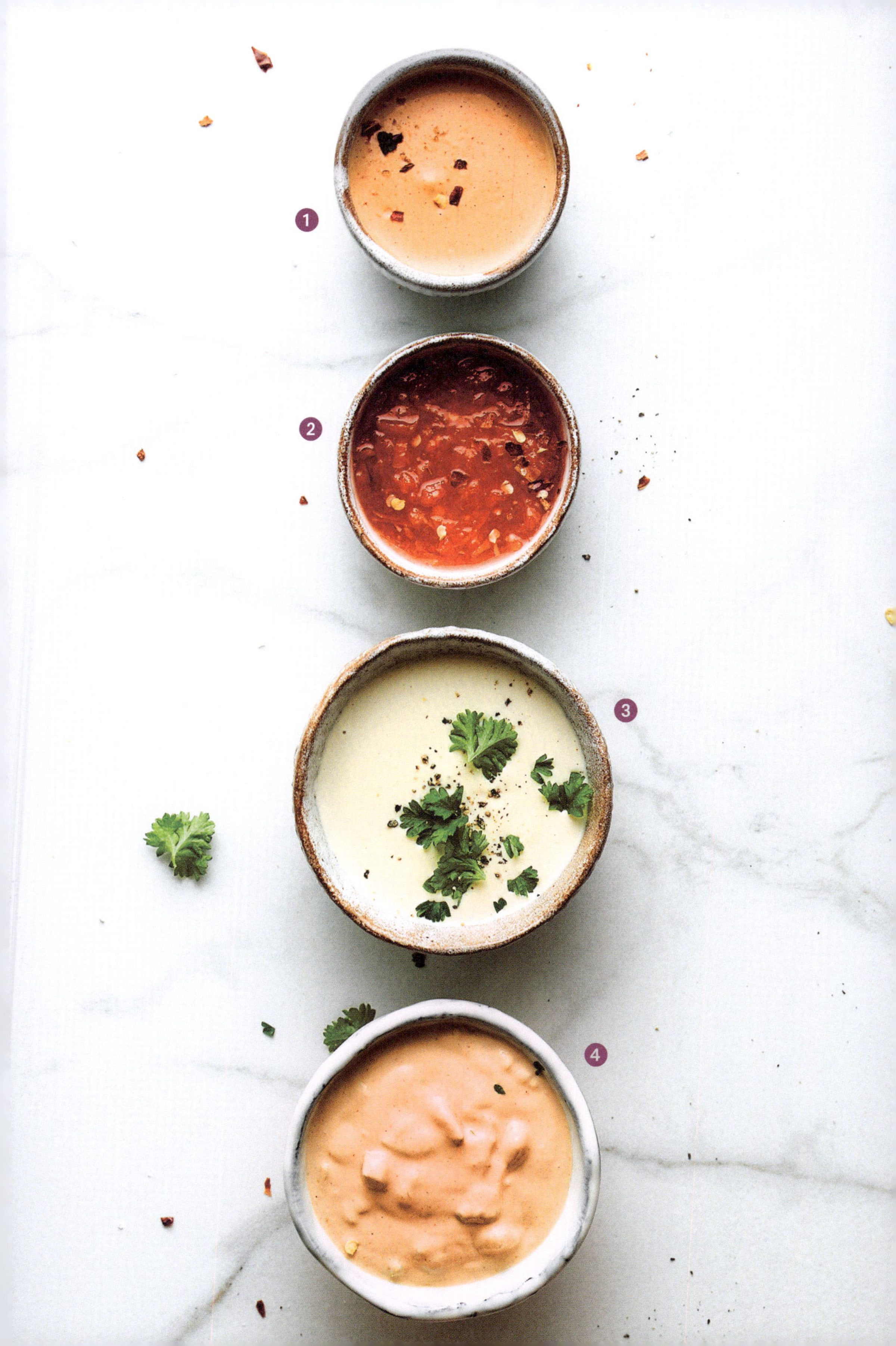
1
2
3
4

SPREAD THE WORD!

4 SIMPLE SPREADS

1 PEA HUMMUS *(makes about 300 ml)*

300 g frozen peas, thawed
1 clove garlic, chopped
2 tbsp tahini (sesame paste)
2 tbsp freshly squeezed lemon juice
½ tsp ground cumin
Sea salt, freshly ground pepper, freshly grated nutmeg

Blend all the ingredients with a stick blender to a creamy but slightly chunky paste. Season with salt, pepper and nutmeg.

2 TANGY HERB CREAM CHEESE
(makes about 250 ml)

200 g cashew nuts, soaked for 4 hours or overnight
75 ml Kanne Brottrunk (fermented bread drink, available online)
1 tbsp freshly squeezed lemon juice
1 clove garlic, crushed
2 tbsp chopped herbs (e.g. chives, parsley)
Sea salt

Drain the soaked cashew nuts in a sieve and transfer to a blender. Add the Brottrunk and lemon juice and blend until smooth. Transfer the mixture to a sterile jar (with as large an opening as possible) and allow to ferment for 48 hours at room temperature, covered with a muslin jar cloth. Then mix the plant-based cream cheese with the remaining ingredients, season with salt and store in an airtight container in the fridge.

3 SUNSHINE CURRY SPREAD
(makes about 250 ml)

80 g sunflower seeds
1 tsp rapeseed oil
1 carrot, finely diced
1 clove garlic, chopped
1 tsp hot curry powder
1 tsp sweet paprika
1 tsp freshly grated ginger
1 tbsp raisins
1 tbsp freshly squeezed lemon juice
Sea salt

Heat a dry non-stick frying pan and toast the sunflower seeds until fragrant. Remove and set aside. Heat 1 tablespoon of oil in a pan and briefly sauté the diced carrot and garlic. Add the sunflower seeds, spices, ginger and raisins and toast the spices for 30 seconds while stirring constantly. Add 150 ml of water and allow to simmer for 5 minutes. Finally, blend everything with a stick blender to a creamy paste and season with the lemon juice and salt.

4 TOMATO HUMMUS *(makes about 300 ml)*

250 g cooked haricot beans
80 g dried tomatoes in oil
2 cloves garlic, chopped
2 tbsp almond butter (or substitute with tahini)
2 tbsp tomato purée
1 tbsp freshly squeezed lemon juice
1 tbsp frozen Italian herbs
Sea salt, freshly ground pepper

Place the beans in a sieve, rinse thoroughly under running water and allow to drain. Remove the tomatoes from the oil, chop and place in a mixing beaker together with all the other ingredients (except the herbs). Blend with a stick blender to a creamy paste. Then gently mix in the herbs and season with salt and pepper.

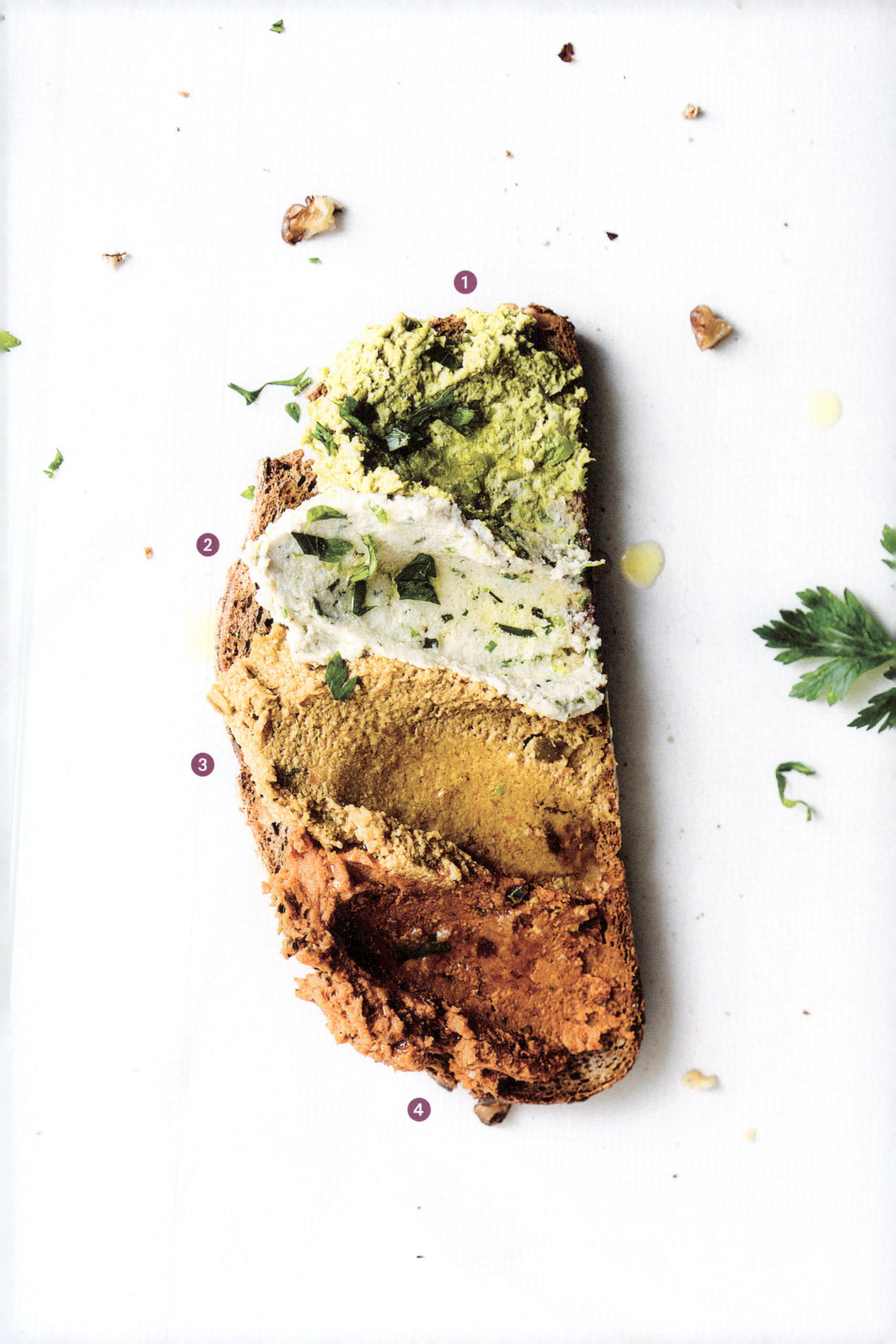
1
2
3
4

RECIPE INDEX

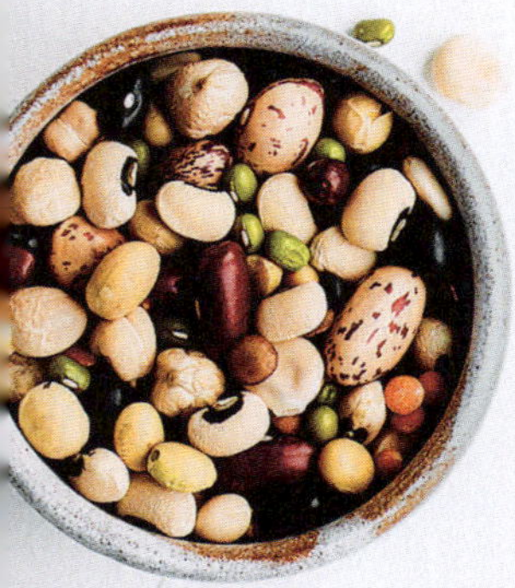

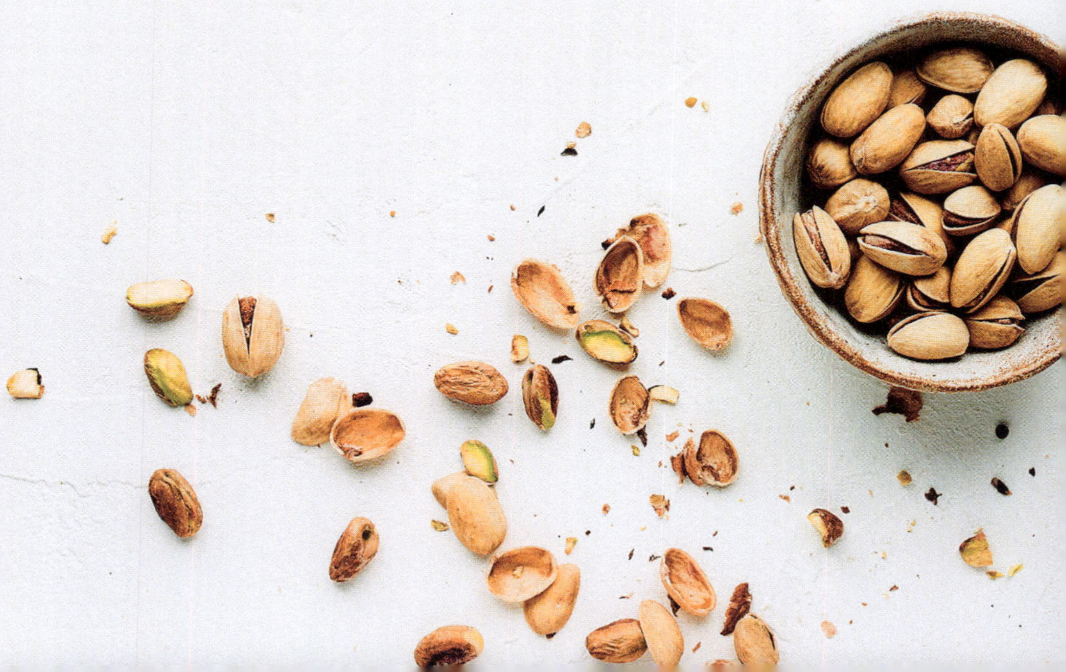

ACKNOWLEDGEMENTS

Although my name is on the cover, this book was only possible thanks to the many people around me who believed in me and accompanied me on this journey. First and foremost, I would like to acknowledge my family, without whose support this project would never have been possible.

Thank you, mum, for putting up with your kitchen and dining room constantly being turned into a battlefield and for helping me clean up after many a wild night of cooking. Your support for me in every endeavour has been unwavering, and I'm eternally grateful to you for that.

Thank you, Dad, for always diligently tasting my creations and helping me to fine-tune the recipes. Without your coffee, those days of work would only have been half as productive.

I thank my two sisters for giving me support and confidence, even and especially in those moments when I felt least able to draw strength from my work.

Thanks to my good friends for always supporting me and never failing to understand my weird notion of time.

Huge thanks go to you all, fabulous readers, Insta-friends and fans of kichererb.se: it was through your support, your many kind words and your great feedback that this book was able to happen in the first place. I feel happy and grateful every day to be able to share what I love doing with you.

Last but not least, my thanks to my publisher and everyone who put their time and energy into bringing this project to fruition. Even now, as I write these lines, I can hardly believe that I am holding my own cookbook in my hands. This is truly a childhood dream come true. THANK YOU.

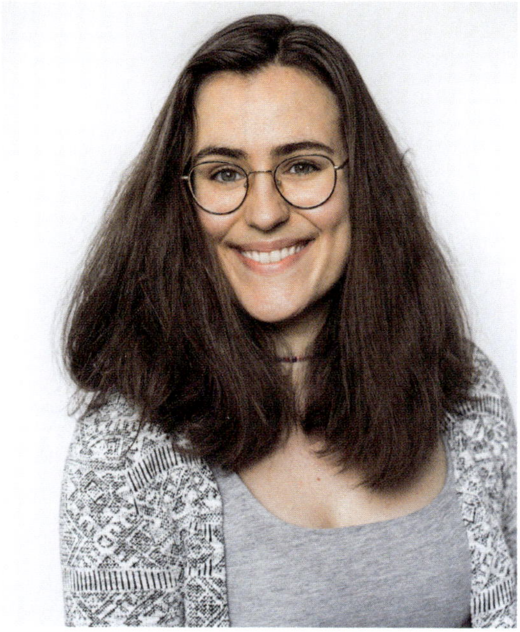

ABOUT THE AUTHOR

Rebekka discovered her passion for cooking at an early age. Having trained as a designer, she combines her love of good food with the creative diversity that comes with both recipe development and photography. Since 2016 she has been running the food blog kichererb.se, where she shares her passion for plant-based cuisine in all its variation and colour. Her main focus is on food that is both filling and makes you happy. *Green Protein* is her first book.

Published in 2026 by Grub Street
4 Rainham Close
London
SW11 6SS

Email: food@grubstreet.co.uk
Web: www.grubstreet.co.uk
X: @grub_street
Facebook: Grub Street Publishing
Instagram: @grubstreet_books

ISBN: 978-1-911714-45-3

A CIP catalogue for this book is available from the British Library.

Published originally in German as Green Protein

Printed and bound by Finidr, Czechia